The Better E

Axel Neustädter is a freelance writer. He edited the gay erotica series *Loverboys*, to which he also contributed three novels. Following his other works, *Gayma Sutra* and the guide to anal sex, *The Bigger Bang*, this book is the latest in his sex manual series published by Bruno Gmünder.

Axel Neustädter

THE BETTER BLOW JOB
Everything You Need to Know About Oral Sex

BRUNO GMÜNDER

We would like to thank Jake Jaxson, RJ Sebastian, and the entire CockyBoys team for the great photos and for being such a pleasure to work with.

THE BETTER BLOW JOB

1st edition
Copyright © 2016 Bruno Gmünder GmbH
Text: © Axel Neustädter
Translation: Nicola Heine

Bruno Gmünder GmbH
Kleiststraße 23-26, 10787 Berlin
info@brunogmuender.com

Cover photos: CockyBoys.com
(Model: Jake Bass)

Printed in Germany

ISBN 978-3-95985-192-3

More about our books and authors:
www.brunogmuender.com

"It's just a penis, right?
Probably no worse for you than smoking."
—*David Sedaris,* When You Are Engulfed in Flames

Author's Note

While I was writing this book, I frequently stopped and asked myself, "Can I really do this? Or am I encouraging risky behavior?" I asked myself this while I was writing the "Seen through a glass" exercise on page 69, for example, or describing the spreader gag on page 105, as well as during the entire chapter on "Swallowing" on page 166. Once you start to worry about these things, leaving the respective passages out always presents itself as a plausible solution—one that I don't agree with at all. Refusing to talk about dumb shit has never stopped anyone from doing it. Not even in bed. So instead, I would like to take this opportunity to make the following point: While most of the actions described in this book are intended for your own personal use, this only applies as long as you're comfortable and don't break anything—whether physically or mentally. If that's too abstract for you, I'll boil it down to this simple and unequivocal formula: Take care of yourselves!

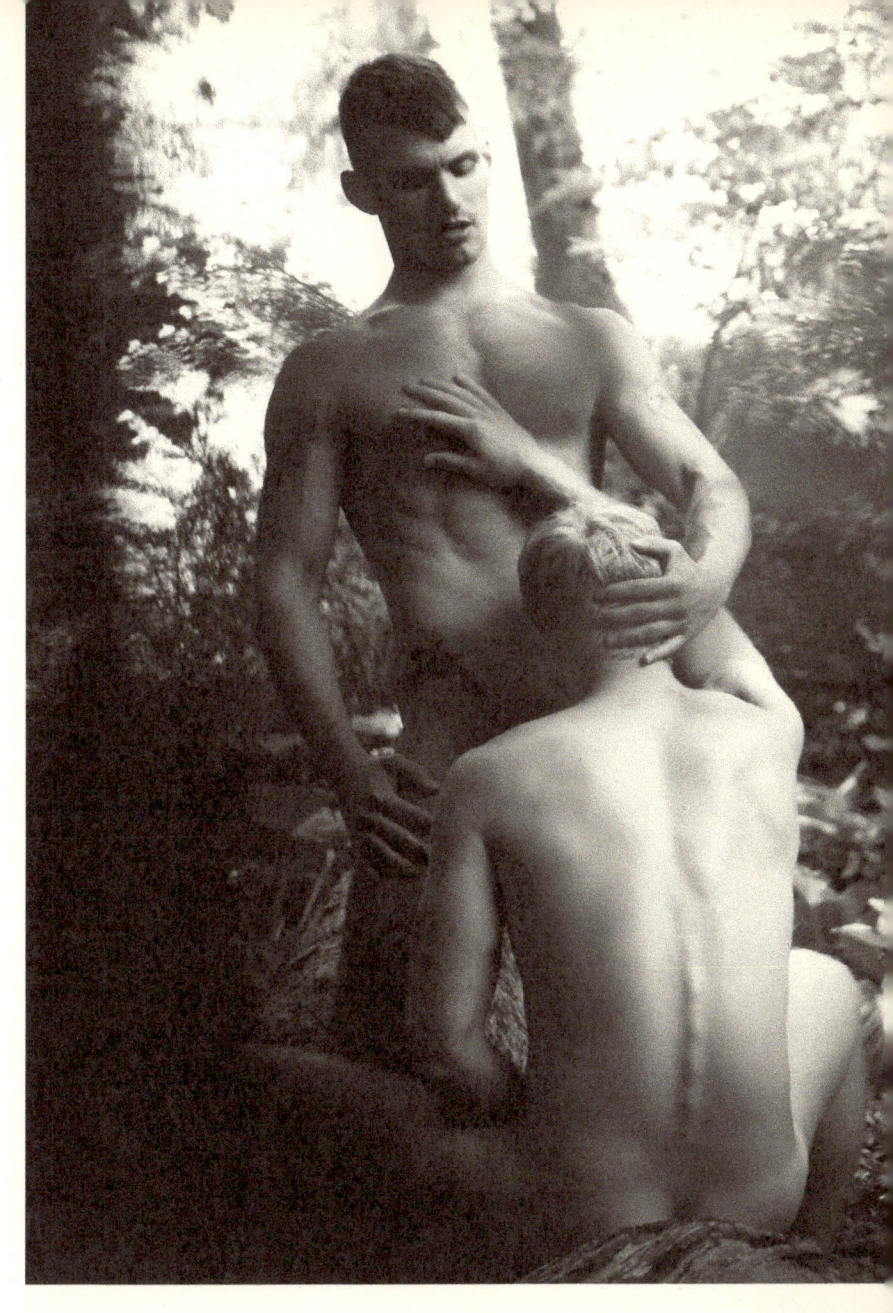

CONTENTS

Preface: Welcome to Blow Job Central 12

TAKE A DEEP BREATH!

Your Genital Socialization 16

French for Beginners—A Basic Guide to Oral Sex................. 20
1 Why "French?" 20
2 Who's the top during oral sex and who's the bottom? 21
3 Are blow jobs "safe?" 21
4 When should you use a lube?................................. 26
5 Why does giving blow jobs make you cry?..................... 28
6 Why is it called a blow job and not a suck job? 29
7 Too small, too big, too clumsy—is there even such a thing?.... 29
8 What are blow job machines good for? 31
9 Are fellatio and cunnilingus the same thing?.................. 33
10 Are there any injury risks involved in oral sex?.............. 34
11 Why does giving someone a blow job make your mouth water?..... 41

Theory Exam: Which Blow Job Department
Is the Best Fit for You? 42

Open Up!

Basic Positions: Taking a Stand.................................. 48

What's Your Blow Job Type? 53
1 Suckers... 53
2 Fluffers... 54
3 Gaggers... 54
4 Swallowers.. 55
5 Lickers.. 56
6 Biters... 57

A Blow Job Artist's Basic Equipment 58

Blow Job Boot Camp for Tops 66
Exercise 1: Frozen Blow Job 68
Exercise 2: Seen Through a Glass 69
Exercise 3: Banana Blow Job 73
Exercise 4: Rubber Bite 75
Exercise 5: Return of the Cucumber 75
Exercise 6: Now You See Me, Now You Don't 77

Get That Dick—How to Do it! 82

Do's & Don'ts When Giving a Blow Job 90

The Triumph of Technique—Blow Job Methods for Tops 93
1 Sloppy Style 93
2 The Gimmick Blow Job 93
3 Lip Service 94
4 The Submissive 96
5 Blind Man's Buff 96
6 Torture 97

Interview with CockyBoys Blow Job Top: Levi Karter 99

Bonus Material: Blow Job Toys for Tops 104
1 Mouth Guard 104
2 Piercings 104
3 Cock Rings 104
4 Blowing Hot and Cold 104
5 Rice, Tic Tacs & Co. 105
6 Food for Thought 105
7 Spreader Gags 105
8 Dildos 107

SHUT YOUR EYES!

Basic Positions: Standing to Attention 110

What's Your Dick Type? 115
1 Humpers 115
2 Jizzers 116
3 Fappers 117
4 Explorers 117
5 Pashas 118
6 Mr. Sensitive 119

Basic Equipment for Receiving a Blow Job 120

Blow Job Boot Camp for Bottoms 130
Exercise 1: The Feather 131
Exercise 2: Wet Dreams 132
Exercise 3: The Melon 135
Exercise 4: Fucking a Glass 136
Exercise 5: Fangs 137
Exercise 6: Blind Faith 137
Exercise 7: Masturbator Action 139

Get That Fuck Mouth—How to Do it! 142

Do's & Don'ts When Receiving a Blow Job 146

The Triumph of Technique: Blow Job Methods for Bottoms 148
1 The Switch 148
2 Live Contest 148
3 Unwrapping 148
4 Extended Play 149
5 Feeding 149
6 Plug Job 149

Interview with CockyBoys Blow Job Bottom: Ricky Roman 151

Bonus Material: Blow Job Gimmicks for Bottoms 156
1 The Portable Hole 156
2 Cock Rings 156
3 Camcorder 156
4 Tattoos & Piercings 157
5 Belts, Ties, Collars 157
6 Water, Water Everywhere 157

RIMMING

From Blow Job to Rim Job 160

Ass-Eating Deluxe—Five Rimming Tips 162
1 Anilingus & Co. 162
2 Cleanliness 163
3 Safer Rimming 164
4 Techniques 165
5 Short & Sweet 165

SWALLOWING

Conspicuous Consumption—A New Phenomenon? 168

Seven Cum Play Techniques, Seven Alternatives 170
1 Swallowing 170
2 Snowballing 170
3 Felching 170
4 Gokkun 171
5 Self-Feeding Yoga 171
6 Chain Reaction 173
7 Semen Doping 173

Shut Your Mouth—Closing Remarks 174

Preface

Welcome to Blow Job Central

Just as fucking is frequently overrated, blow jobs are often underrated. Which provides an answer to the completely understandable question as to why, after writing a guide to *The Bigger Bang*, I suddenly decided to dial it down a notch and devote an entire book to the subject of blow jobs. But there's another reason why I pestered my editor to let me write this book: First of all, in my experience, oral sex is ideally suited to today's culture of dating apps and YouPorn. And secondly, it's becoming increasingly more important.

At the time of writing, the search terms "suck" and "fuck" both rack up around 600 hits each on Manhunt, while "blow job" scores only around 201 hits. OK, that doesn't tell us much. But if you consider that a British "Sexual Health" survey conducted in 2012 showed that oral sex was the most common sexual practice among men who have sex with men (with mutual masturbation in second place and anal sex coming third), while according to a survey conducted in the United States in 2011, the ratio between oral sex and anal sex was 72.7 percent to 37.2 percent, this sheds an entirely different light on the matter. In addition, the immense proliferation of blow job websites such as SuckOffGuys.com or CumPigMen.com is undeniable. Even established porn studios such as Fratmen or Treasure Island have long since created designated channels for "cocksucking" aficionados. Admittedly, these are devoted not only to the glorification of sucking dick, but also to the fetishization of jizz and swallowing semen. The eternal fascination with the "brojob" phenomenon (playfully "milking" a straight guy so sexually starved, he willingly submits to being serviced by either a fellow sufferer or a willing gay man) also plays a large role. But all of these are just additional reasons for taking a closer, more critical look at the topic of the blow job in all its aspects.

My own main concern when writing this book was to encourage my readers to reassess their own needs and to create a greater awareness for blow jobs as a fully-fledged sex act. There is a reason for this. When I'm on a date, I frequently get the feeling that some guys just go through the motions of a blow job superficially and without concentrating properly, because they feel they need to save up their erectile energy for fucking later on. That's understandable enough. If you've hooked up with another guy to fuck, you don't want to literally blow your load beforehand. On the other hand: I've seen plenty of dicks where a cursory and hurried suck and gulp would be a terrible waste. And often enough, these dicks are attached to guys who appreciate a dedicated blow job far more than a hasty fuck. So there's no need to let your sense of duty rob you of your own pleasure. Or to put it bluntly: A fully savored blow job is far better than a half-hearted suck'n'fuck session. Besides, it may be simply a lack of experience that prevents you from savoring the act. Blow jobs, whether you're giving or receiving, require skill—and this can be learned. So let us view the first three sections of this book as a basic how-to guide, while the last two were written with the more advanced practitioners in mind. If this results in one reader or another rediscovering the joys of a sex act that habit and routine have turned into a pit-stop on the road to the main act, I will consider my job done. And if you're already a blow job addict, you'll find plenty to enjoy either way.

> *Oral is more popular among guys than anal, with a ratio of 72 to 37 percent.*

So shut your eyes, open your mouth and... start reading!

Axel Neustädter

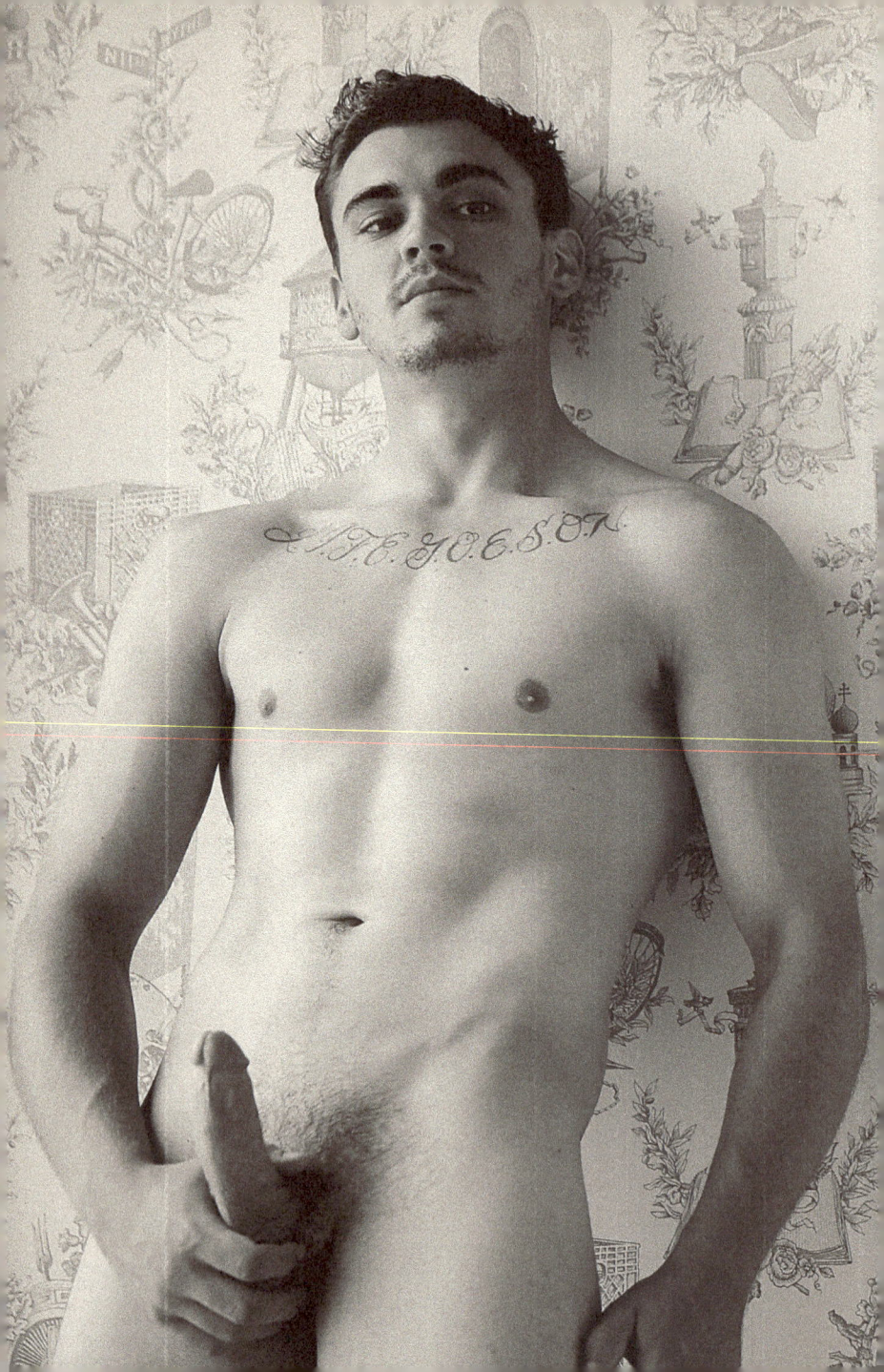

TAKE A DEEP BREATH!
Dick Meets Mouth

Take a Deep Breath!

Your Genital Socialization

But before we start blowing anyone else, let's blow up our own egos. After all, it's just us here. And we're all champions. Because every man is a natural born blow job artist.

Now I've probably just raised a hollow laugh from those of you who have wasted any number of dates on an inept blow job provider. And I'll have hopefully raised a laugh among the inept blow job providers themselves, who are aware of their shortcomings, without being bitter about them. After all, if you're going to make fun of a bungled blow job, you should prove that you're better at it yourself. And eradicating shortcomings is what we're here for. So first of all, let's just take a moment to appreciate the immense privilege that man-on-man fellatio affords us. Unlike male-female pairings, gay blow jobs involve two partners who have had their entire lives to familiarize themselves with dicks. Not only in theory, but in practice as well. Because all of them have their own personal dick.

Some of you might object to being included in the dick-worshipping faction, as you're more into asses. Or into lips and mouths, which would be another excellent reason for reading this book. That may well be the case. Nevertheless, I stand by my claim: However fixated on asses, lips or mouths you may be, this doesn't change the fact that every gay man has, in the course of exploring his sexuality, at some point engaged with his own penis. This is due to the three steps of what I'd like to call "genital socialization."

▼ Step One

Even if you've never shown much interest in your pee-pee as a child, you will probably have gotten to know it during your first forays into masturbation.

▼ Step Two

While your own masturbatory practices can very quickly settle into a rut, first sexual encounters with other people will force you to question the quality and functionality of your own wang.

▼ Step Three

As soon as you start exploring gay infrastructures (even if it's just dating sites), you are generally confronted with the eternal tug-of-war between cock hunger and cock presentation. Which is another reason to reassess the relationship between you and your dick.

Some people experience these three steps consciously, others less so, but the fact remains that they are all steps in the development of every man's relationship with his penis. It's a bit like how friendships work. First you get to know each other, and then you go through situations that test your mutual loyalty before finally discovering how compatible you both are with the rest of the gay community.

> *The relationship between a man and his dick can be amicable or hostile.*

The amicability of your relationship will depend largely on how smoothly you pass through the individual steps. Your relationship may be amicable or it may be hostile. But either way, it will have a profound effect on your relationship with other men's dicks.

If you have an exceptionally close relationship with your own dick, you'll be able to fine-tune its optimal "care" over time, while if your relationship with your schlong is just average or even below average, then you'll probably tend to concentrate on "servicing" the other man's penis to the best of your ability. Oh dear, did I really just say "the other man's penis"? Surely that's what married women call their lover's junk, isn't it? Oh well, the term works just as well here.

Getting back to the privilege of being a natural born blow job artist: Just because step three of your genital socialization generally results in a subdivision of servicers and servicees, that shouldn't stop you from revisiting steps one and two any time you like. If your blow job skills stagnate, a closer inspection of your own boner can help you explore other ways of showing it a good time. And if you hit a wall when optimizing your own methods of stimulation, you can just switch sides and find out what kind of treatment another guy's cock will respond to. Ideally of course, this exchange should take place all the time. After all, there's a reason that the famous 69 position, which involves both partners sucking each other's dicks simultaneously, is widely considered the ultimate romantic ideal. We might add a fourth step as the ultimate objective of every man's genital socialization—namely taking the same amount of pleasure in fulfilling and enjoying both roles. Thanks to your privileged vantage point: Looking back on years of experience with your own and other people's dicks, this is not an unrealistic goal. But for the time being, let's concentrate on putting an end to all the inept blow jobs on this planet. For this purpose, we will start out by clearing a few basic principles concerning the sexual practice commonly known as "French." Why is that? Turn the page, champ!

> *The final goal of your genital socialization should be the 69 position.*

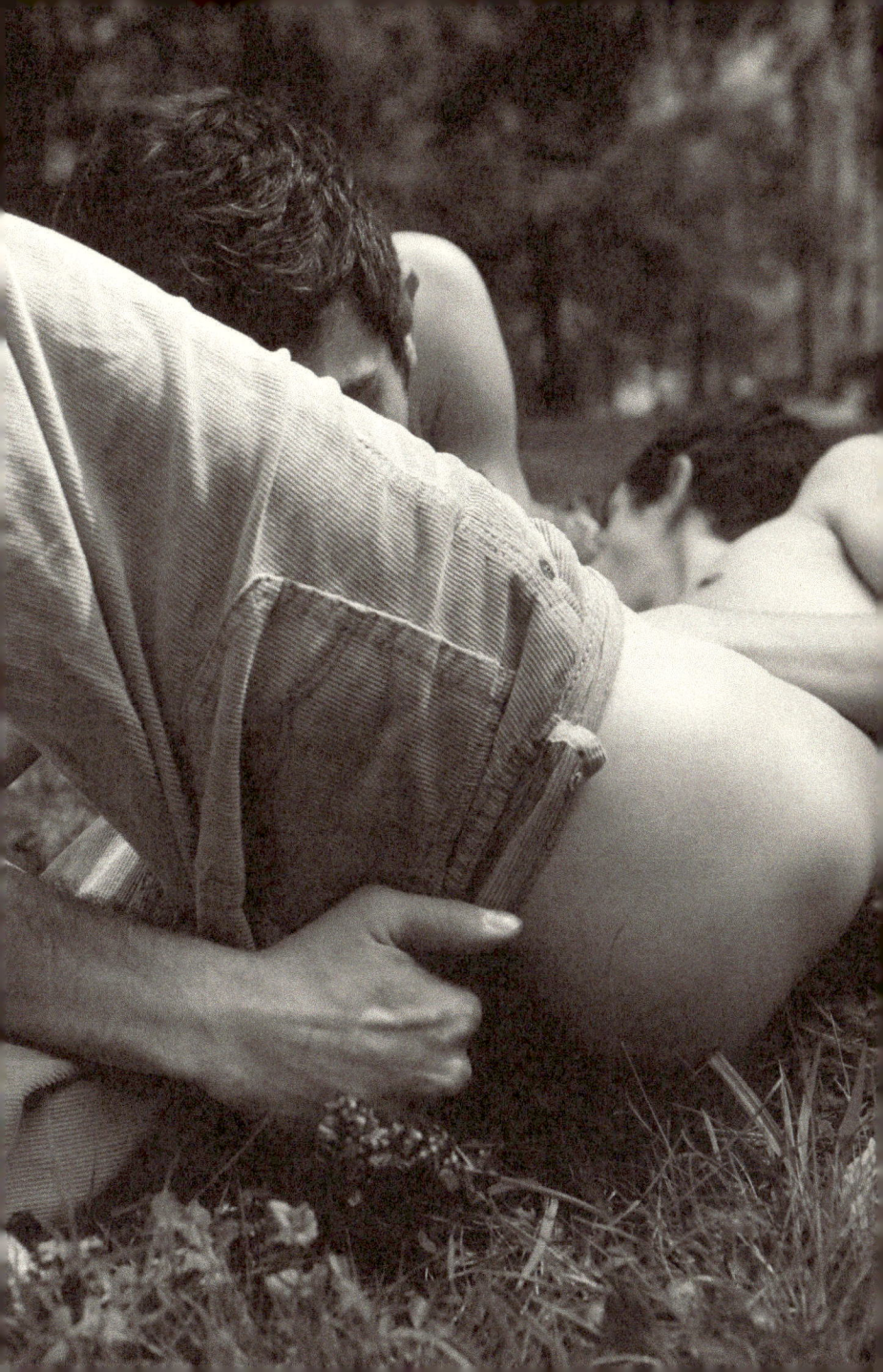

French for Beginners—A Basic Guide to Oral Sex

▼ Why "French?"

This question is as banal as it is tricky—because it has not one answer, but several. In my opinion, none of them are entirely convincing. Feel free to choose whichever of the more common explanations you like best. We'll start simple and get more sophisticated as we proceed.

Theory 1: The only reason it's called that is because Greek, Spanish, English, and German were already reserved for anal, tit fucking, "kneepit" sex, and missionary.

Theory 2: Paris is the city of love and, France being a highly centralized country, represents the entire nation. Which is why a lovingly given blow job was known as French sex.

Theory 3: Fellatio is the most popular sex act among the French, a claim whose veracity was actually confirmed by the "Enquête sur la sexualité en France" in 2008.

Theory 4: Just as in Islamic countries today, oral sex was not exactly prohibited but still frowned upon in western cultures up until the twentieth century. As the British Empire's sworn enemy was France and its "decadent" capital Paris had always had the reputation of being extremely lax, the term "French" was used pejoratively to bring oral sex into discredit.

Theory 5: In the Middle Ages, syphilis was known as the "French disease." It led to many prostitutes restricting their services to oral sex as a means of prevention. As we will see later, this protective measure was completely pointless. But it may have led to oral sex being seen as a "French" specialty.

▼ Who's the top during oral sex and who's the bottom?

One of the blow job's more distinctive revolutionary qualities is that it turns traditional bottom and top roles upside down. The question of who takes on which role during oral sex has had me confused for years. But now I use the following rule of thumb: Most blow job tops are anal bottoms.

That is to say: If you're into sucking dicks, you probably don't mind having them shoved up your backside. A bottom cliché with a top half, so to speak. This definition is based on the assumption that engulfing a dick in your mouth is an act of taking, while doing the same thing with your ass is an act of being taken. Whether this is always the case in practice is of course debatable—but to avoid misunderstandings, this is the definition I'm going to use for this book. So to put it succinctly: cocksucker = top, blow job receiver = bottom.

▼ Are blow jobs "safe?"

They are not. For even though it is relatively unlikely that you will infect someone with HIV via a blow job, there are a host of other sexually transmitted infections that can be easily shared via oral sex. The most important of these being herpes, hepatitis B, gonorrhea, and syphilis. I'll go into protective measures shortly, but for now, here is a brief overview.

Herpes: Herpes simplex causes tiny, itchy, burning blisters that burst under pressure and ooze infectious fluids. They can appear on your lips and mouth as well as around your genitals and anus. There are two different types of herpes (oral and genital), which share some of the same characteristics. Oral herpes can facilitate a genital herpes infection. The virus is transmitted by the fluid from open herpes blisters coming into contact with your mouth, dick, or anus. A herpes infection is not essentially an enormous tragedy (estimates suggest that 90 percent of adults carry the oral herpes virus, although only one in three or four people actually have any symptoms), but it does weaken the immune system and it is incurable. If you have ever been infected with herpes, there is always a chance of stress, disgust, or illness causing the blisters to reappear. Special creams available from the drugstore can accelerate the healing process, or you can just let them heal up on their own.

Hepatitis B: Of all the hepatitis viruses, a group of nasty diseases that cause liver infections, Type B is the most infectious (transmitted via blood, semen, and saliva). On the other hand, it is comparatively harmless and clears up on its own in 90 percent of cases. Only 5 to 10 percent of cases result in a chronic infection, leading to lasting liver damage. You can and should avoid this risk in the first place by getting yourself vaccinated. Hepatitis vaccinations involve two, sometimes three injections administered one to two months apart. After that, you will generally be immune to the virus. Being gay means that you are officially at risk of contracting the disease, so the vaccine is free in most countries. You should also take the opportunity of getting yourself vaccinated against hepatitis A as well (which is frequently transmitted via rimming).

Gonorrhea: Symptoms of a gonorrhea infection (also known as the clap), which affects the urethra in particular, include pain and discharge. If left untreated, it can lead to inflammation of the prostate and the epididymis and even infertility. If you engage in unprotected anal or oral intercourse, it can also affect the region around the anus or the throat. So if you suffer from pain while urinating or defecating, or if you notice a discharge, see your doctor at once and ask for a swab test. Gonorrhea can be treated quickly and easily with antibiotics, but a vaccine against the infection is currently not available.

You can contract gonorrhea of the throat via oral sex.

Syphilis: Similar to herpes but much more severe, the first signs of syphilis are lesions in and around the penis, the anus, or the mouth. Contact with these lesions, especially if they ooze fluid, is highly infectious. A couple of weeks after they have healed, you'll be hit by the second stage of the disease, with fever and rashes all over your skin. It is highly contagious during this stage is well. After that, you'll feel better for a while, for years even. But all this time, the infection will continue to rage inside you, attacking your internal organs and cardiovascular system, your bone structure, your brain, and your nervous system. If left untreated, the consequences can be deadly. So if you have even the slightest cause to suspect you might have picked up syphilis, see your doctor right away and ask for a blood test! It can be cured entirely with penicillin if administered in time.

> *Talking about STIs always raises the sex-negativity alarm, right?*

So that's enough of that! I can't deny that anytime I have to list and describe sexually transmitted diseases and their symptoms, I start to worry about sounding sex-negative. After all, at first glance, this kind of information has a highly off-putting and, as a consequence, boner-killing effect, right? But only at first glance. Ultimately, it's a question of educating yourself about the risks and recognizing the liberating qualities of informed action.

It's quite simple really: Pretty much every man taking his first tentative steps into the gay scene will sooner or later be confronted with the fear of having caught some sexually transmitted infection or other—whether following a quick and dirty hookup with a stranger, a broken condom, or after getting carried away and omitting to use a condom at all. The mother of all fears, even today, when combined Anti-Retroviral Therapy is freely available in most parts, is experienced daily by hundreds of gay men all over the world applying for PEP (post-exposure prophylaxis) after unsafe sex, or waiting for their HIV test results. We encounter a more abstract version of this fear during those confusing moments during a date or an anonymous hookup, when you suddenly realize that you're no longer sure whether you've just entered the danger zone. This kind of thing happens more frequently in situations where a less experienced guy hooks up with a more experienced partner who encourages him to do stuff he's never even considered before. In cases such as these, the best answer is always "I'll do it once I've educated myself about what I'm getting myself into." But in real life, confusion often leads to a loss of confidence and many men end up just going along with it. After all, no one wants to look like a complete newbie. And no one wants to be a party pooper. This is exacerbated by the fact that horniness tends to crowd out any fears or inhibitions. So you just go with it and hope for the best. Only to find yourself panicking afterwards, as described above. It's a real predicament.

> *No one wants to come across as a total newbie.*

What I'm trying to point out is: The better informed you are, the less likely you are to run into these moments of confusion. If you know what you want and know what you're doing, it's a lot easier to avoid getting talked into doing something you'll regret later on. So if you're one of those guys who starts rolling their eyes and skipping ahead to the next part as soon as they read the words "sexually transmitted infection," then please get this straight: Educating yourself will save you a lot of stress, increase your sexual autonomy, and liberate your sex life. So please, take another look at the pages you skipped over, man up, and take a proper look at the risks. It's better to encounter them theoretically, however reluctantly, than to have to deal with them in practice. Apart from that, make your blow jobs as safe as possible by sticking to the following rules.

Six Rules for Safer Blow Jobs

1. *Never wrap your lips around a dick that exhibits the visual signs of any of the aforementioned infections, and never stick your dick into a mouth that does this either.*

2. *If you are not sure whether or not you have an infection, play fair and don't engage in any sexual activities until you've consulted your doctor. Don't start having sex again until you're absolutely sure you won't infect your partner.*

3. *If you only feel comfortable having oral sex with a condom, that's fine, but you do need to let your partner know beforehand. This will save you both potential embarrassment and buzzkill. In my experience, neither tops nor bottoms have a clear majority for preferring blow jobs with a condom.*

4. *Accept this fundamental truth: There is no such thing as completely safe sex. So there is no point in trusting in the belief that you have done all the right things. If you have any doubts about your health, see a doctor and, until you do, abide by rule number 2.*

5. *Are you HIV-positive, or are you planning on messing around with someone who is? As I mentioned earlier, being HIV-positive is not a problem for oral sex—in principle. Especially if the positive partner is non-viremic. Nevertheless, please play close attention to rule 6 in particular!*

6. *Are you into cum swallowing? Here's the good news: You are not alone—far from it. The bad news: Swallowing is by far the least safe aspect of oral sex. So before you become a habitual cum swallower, please read the entire chapter on "Swallowing" on page 166.*

▼ When should you use a lube?

In most cases, your own naturally produced saliva (which is activated when you perform a blow job) should be enough to reduce friction for both the top and the bottom. If you do want to use a lube as well, read the packaging or instruction leaflet first. If these state "For external use only" or "Not for human consumption," you will need to find an alternative. Substances such as Crisco or Vaseline, which are sometimes used for anal sex without a condom (as these attack the latex) are not recommended for oral use, as they may contain mineral oils. Besides, they are rarely moist enough to be much use. Silicone-based lubes have not been proven to be harmful, but water-based lubes are a better choice—these are also available in a range of artificial flavors. Possible reasons for using a lube:

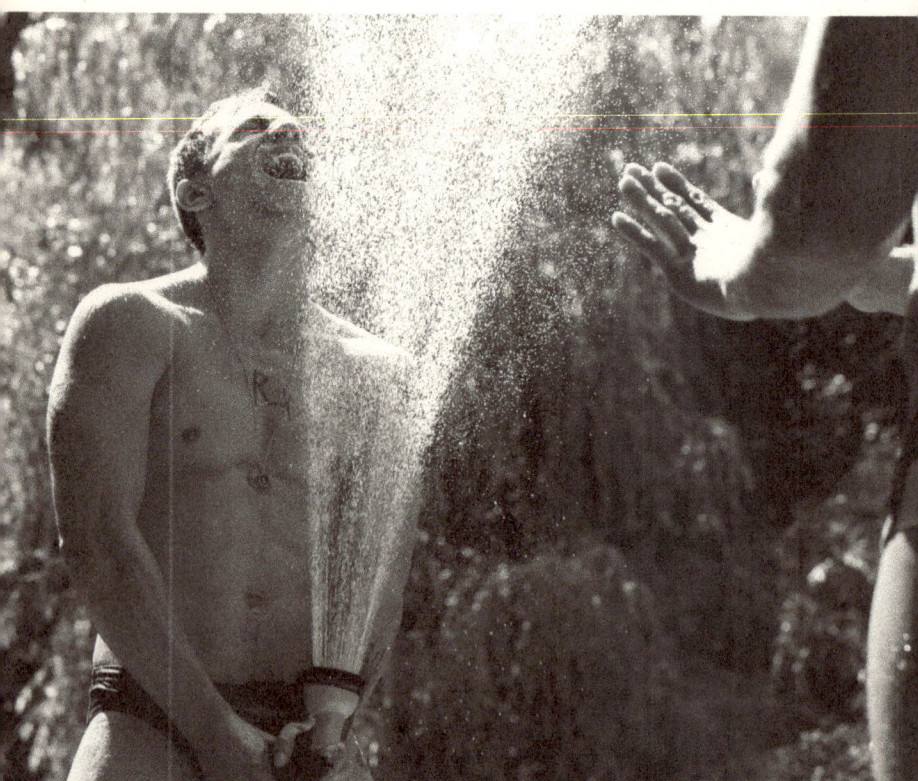

A) A dry mouth/chapped lips on the part of the top
B) Extreme sensitivity to touch on the part of the bottom
C) For the sake of variety and experimentation
D) An aversion to the taste of dick

So far, so objective. But I can't just let that go without a few comments of my own.

Reason D: If you really need to smother the taste of your partner's dick with synthetically flavored lube to be able to enjoy oral sex, you might want to either tell your guy to take a shower or just stop giving blow jobs altogether. If your erotic attraction is impaired on such a fundamental level, I really don't see how you can enjoy having sex at all.

Reason C: If curiosity, rather that desperation, leads you to rummage around in the stock of sex aids, you'll find plenty of variety. The list of available flavorings ranges from the classic strawberry and banana, to party flavors such as champagne and piña colada and even festive Christmas editions flavored with marzipan. Personally, I think they're all gross and pointless, but fortunately, that is purely a matter of taste.

Reason B: If you're forced to use lube to reduce friction due to the sensitivity of your partner's genitals, you might want to take a closer look at your own blow job technique. This is especially advisable if you have no or only a few previous partners as a basis for comparison. Should you attempt to cure your partner's hypersensitivity with "desensitizing" (translation: numbing) creams, please remember that these will affect your mouth as well. Always check for allergies and intolerance before using them!

Reason A: Dry mouth (the medical term is xerostomia) may have a variety of causes—from nervousness about the possible side effects of medication to the original ailment itself. Chronic dry mouth can be alleviated by using synthetic saliva sprays available over the counter from most pharmacies. Home remedies include: drinking plenty, chewing gum, or sucking candy. Remember to take the candy out of your mouth before oral sex! Chapped lips and cracks at the corners of your mouth can be prevented by using lip balm or applying honey or olive oil before bed.

▼ Why does giving blow jobs make you cry?

Some of my readers may not understand the question, but anyone who has ever tried to perform an extensive deep-throat blow job will know exactly what I mean. Having a dick thrust repeatedly far down your throat will make your eyes water and your nose run at some point. The romantic explanation for this response is "some dicks are so beautiful, they'll make you cry," but it's rarely meant seriously and is, of course, complete nonsense. The unromantic truth is that this reaction is caused by the gag reflex activated by a deep blow job.

This is an entirely normal bodily reaction: a foreign body threatening to penetrate the trachea causes the pharynx to contract. That's what's making you gag. If this happens several times in succession, the strain and attendant pressure leads to an increased production of fluid in your tear ducts. While the average quantity of tear fluid is produced simply to keep the retina moist, the surplus being drained off through the nose, where it evaporates, an above average quantity will drain off via the eyes as well.

> *Do blow jobs make you cry "emotional tears" or "reflex tears"?*

This is what's making you cry. There's a difference between "reflex tears" and "emotional tears." The latter contain more proteins, potassium and the happiness hormone serotonin. Whether blow jobs produce reflex tears or emotional ones has, to the best of my knowledge, never been analyzed. The burden of proof for weeping over a blow job being an expression of your feelings lies with the romantics. Until they prove otherwise, the cry reflex is supported by the following rather distasteful, but entirely reasonable, comparison: Throwing up makes your eyes water too.

▼ Why is it called a blow job and not a suck job?

Nobody really knows how the term "blow," which could give rise to terrible misunderstandings, became an established label for oral sex. On the other hand, everyone knows it's complete crapola. No one has ever attempted to actually blow up another guy's dick. At least, no on who actually likes their partner. The correct term would of course be "suck job." Nevertheless, the term "blow" is an international phenomenon. The Germans call it "blasen" (blow), the Dutch prefer the term "pijpbeurt" (literally "pipe turn"), the Italians do the "pompino" (little pump) and the French go with "pipe." One theory postulates that all these cutesy terms stem back to a time when sex was a taboo subject and if you did have to talk about it, shame and embarrassment led you to fall back on metaphors and double entendre. Sounds fairly plausible. But that doesn't answer the question of why we're still stuck with these metaphors in these times of TMI frankness. Our terminology used to be far more direct, as demonstrated by the Latin term "fellatio," which is derived from the verb "fellare"—"to suck." It just goes to show how much more civilized the ancient Romans were in many respects.

▼ Too small, too big, too clumsy—
is there even such a thing?

Earlier on, we discussed the "inept" blow job, whose practitioners would presumably fall into the category "too clumsy." But to be honest: Of the three qualities in the subheading, "too clumsy" is the only one of which I can categorically state that does not exist. Clumsiness is—with a lot of practice—curable, and even if you have no motors skills whatsoever, with the right kind of training, you can still be a real blow job artist. See the following pages for training tips. That leaves us with "too small" and "too big"—both of which can be applied, in the context of oral sex, to both mouths and dicks. In this regard, the jury is split by 2 to 2.

Your dick is too big: Generally, even the most impressive wang will find a suitable mouth, but in some cases, the bottom's dick may well be too large for his partner's mouth. That doesn't mean you need to throw in the towel, so to speak. The top may still be able to suck the bottom's glans, and then finish him off with a combination of licking, jerking off, massage, and plenty of spit. A good blow job is not just a bout of mouth fucking to the exclusion of everything else, and it does not have to involve deep-throating. See the section on "Working Materials" in the chapter "Open Your Mouth" for further suggestions.

Your mouth is too small: If a dick can be too large for a blow job, then logically, some mouths may be too small. Cases of the actual mouth opening being too small are relatively rare. This is because the skin around your mouth is elastic and you can expand the opening simply by using your finger to stretch it. But then there's the jaw, the oral cavity, and the throat. The size and capacity of these parts of your anatomy can in fact vary enormously. If you can't give a guy a blow job without your teeth scraping his boner, oral sex is going to be a fucking chore for both of you. Again, see the section on "Working Materials" in the chapter "Open Your Mouth" for suggestions.

Your dick's too small: That doesn't even make sense. Of course, in some rare cases you may come across a micropenis which will admittedly fail to fill up your mouth, but that doesn't mean you can't suck it. You'll just have to be a bit more careful and pay more attention to detail. In this case, "careful" refers to targeted stimulation of a smaller area. Equating a lack of size with fragility or hypersensitivity is simply nonsense. If it does hurt, your bottom will let you know.

Your mouth's too big: Does not apply either. Even if your mouth is enormous, you should still be able to purse your lips, and even the largest oral cavity has boundaries that provide friction for any dick. If a full-house feeling is that important to you, you're just going to have to swallow several dicks at once. You shouldn't have any trouble finding a couple of volunteers!

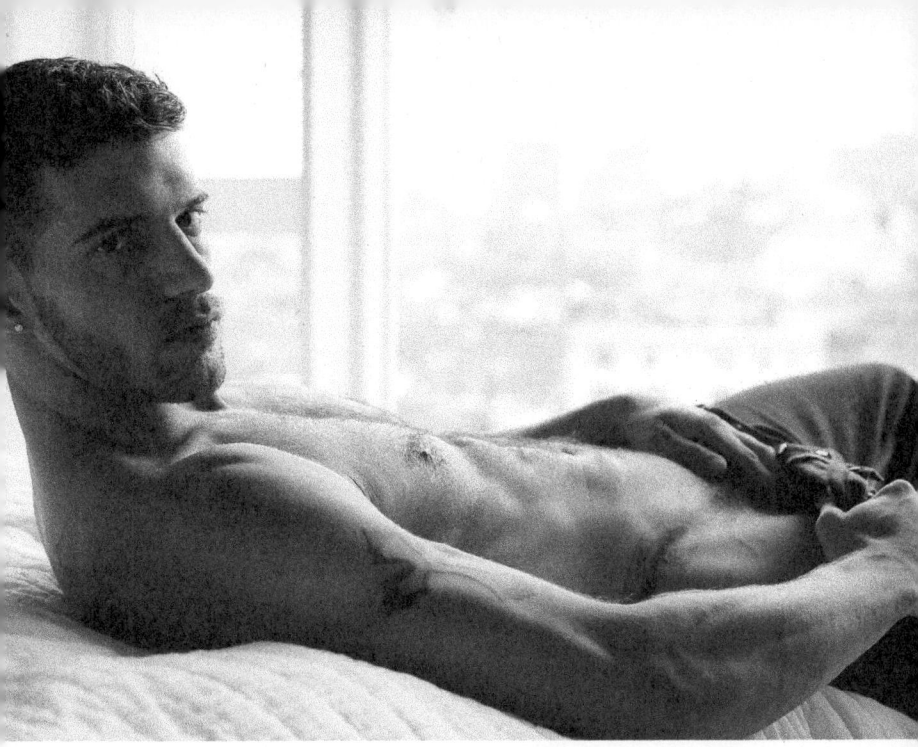

▼ What are blow job machines good for?

The Internet hype surrounding the launch of the Autoblow 2 in the spring of 2014 was a sign of the general fascination surrounding oral sex—even if it is performed by a machine.

Some background information: In the spring of that year, lawyer Brian Sloan started an Indiegogo crowdfunding campaign to raise $45,000 towards manufacturing a newly invented product called the Autoblow 2. Unlike most masturbators currently on the market, this cylindrical gadget featured not only tubular silicon mouths in three sizes with any amount of lube, but also a motorized stimulation coil that moved back and forth underneath the silicon tubes at three, individually set speeds. In other words: Once you stuck your boner inside the lubed up tube and switched the machine on, you were greeted with a rhythmic up and down movement that imitated the sucking motion of a real mouth "extraordinarily well." Straight to the dumpster? No way. The thing became an overnight sensation. When a month had passed and the campaign was over, thousands of donors had funded the project to the tune of over $280,00, way more than the $45,000 target, and when just a little while later the Autoblow website switched to pre-order mode, it promptly crashed under the sheer demand. Since then, Sloan has expanded his product line (to include a prostate stimulator guaranteed to buzz your P-spot) and is still raking in a ridiculous of cash in Autoblow 2 sales—just as the manufacturers of more established masturbators such as Fleshlight or Venga have been doing for years. Clearly, blow job machines are popular among a wide range of consumers. So there is no need to be embarrassed for using them, or at least, no reason not to try them out. But in order to answer our opening question, we're going to have to go into more detail. It really depends on what you're hoping to get from the machine. Six Points to Consider:

1 You like giving blow jobs and you want to use the machine to improve your technique.
Forget it. You can't learn technique from technology.

2 You want to practice with the machine before a real live person gives you your first blow job.
Don't. Communication and responding to the guy providing the blow job are essential duties of the person receiving. You're more likely to blunt these skills with a machine than hone them.

3 You always cum too quickly whenever someone gives you a blow job and you want to use the machine to "toughen yourself up."
Why not? It's worth a try. Just one word of warning: Don't hang your hopes in this method too high. It is one thing to stay in control in the comfort of your own room, enjoying the steady, repetitive motion of a machine—and quite another to resist the "unpredictable" oral skills of a real live partner who really turns you on.

4 As a blow job bottom you're tired of having your dick sucked by all these delicate flowers, and you're looking for a replacement.
Let me put it this way: According to Brian Sloan, the Autoblow 2 engine can keep going for up to 1,000 hours. This means that it can provide you with a 42-day blow job without stopping. You're not going to find a human being who can do that. So if superhuman endurance and constant readiness are more important to you than human interaction and eroticism, then maybe you would be better off with a machine. But don't let your social skills wither away in the process.

5 You want to blow and be blown at the same time. So you and your boyfriend are hooking up with a machine.
It's a fun idea in theory, but too much like hard work in practice. The first challenge consists of finding the right position where you're more or less in control of the masturbator (having your partner lie flat on his back with you on top of him and the machine underneath you works quite well), and the machine's monotonous rhythm and the pretty loud rattling sound can make it hard to concentrate. The 69 position is a simpler and better strategy for simultaneous oral.

6 You just want to add a little variety to your masturbatory repertoire.
There it is: The only really good reason for getting yourself a blow job machine.

▼ Are fellatio and cunnilingus the same thing?

They are not. While fellatio refers to orally pleasuring the penis, cunnilingus means licking the female genitalia (Latin "cunnus"). If your sexual encounters involve two guys with dicks, cunnilingus simply isn't going to be an option. But if cunnilingus has somehow found its way onto your sexual to-do list, even though you're not interested in heterosexual sex, you can try replacing it with "analingus"—rimming—instead. That works just as well with either sex.

▼ Are there any injury risks involved in oral sex?

We went into all the major infection risks when we answered the question of whether oral sex is safe, so now it's time to take a look at actual blow job accidents. Most of these, while frequently overly hyped, hardly ever occur in real life. I'll go into them briefly nonetheless, if only to make them less scary. Essentially, the risk of injury involved in oral sex is fairly low. As long as you stick to the "Topping During Oral Sex: Don'ts" on page 91/147, you have pretty much nothing to fear. The rest is a matter of luck, as only abstinence can give you a hundred percent protection. And that's not what we're here for. So take a deep breath—we'll get through this together!

INJURY RISKS FOR TOPS

Fainting and Asphyxiation

Some of you may remember blow job expert Lara Love's failed attempt at setting a world record for giving head. In January 2011, the twenty-three-year-old starlet tried to suck off 250 guys to orgasm, but was forced to quit after Mr. 150 because she kept blacking out. In my opinion, the absurd dimensions of this scenario are a pretty good indication of how likely you are to lose consciousness while giving someone a blow job. You really do have to go to ridiculous lengths before you reach that point. Besides, if silly little Miss Love managed to listen to what her body was telling her before actually breaking down, you should certainly be able to. So if you hyperventilate, keep an eye on your breathing. And if you start feeling nauseous or dizzy, let your partner know, and take a break. As far as asphyxiation is concerned, breath-play, as enjoyed by advanced BDSM practitioners, often involves holding someone's nose while they deep throat you. This can indeed stop you from sucking air. But as I said, this is reserved for experienced practitioners who are aware that BDSM play requires some practice and a lot of trust and responsibility. It definitely does not happen "accidentally."

Tearing the Corners of Your Mouth

Less harmful, but more realistic: If your lips are dry or chapped, opening your mouth—which you're going to have to do if you're sucking someone off—can lead to you tearing the skin at the corners of your mouth. This is harmless, but still pretty unpleasant, so you should take steps to prevent it. Dry skin around your mouth can be caused, for example, by an iron or zinc deficiency, both of which can be remedied by eating spinach, porridge oats, eggs, or cheese. Skin creams and lip balm can also help your skin regain its elasticity. If you've already torn the corners of your mouth, you should avoid opening it wide for the time being. Repeated tearing of the affected areas can lead to unpleasant infections. In addition, it can also contribute to infections such as herpes (which can also be a cause of tearing themselves).

A Dislocated Jaw

If your jaw isn't already damaged in some way, it's highly unlikely that giving a blow job will cause dislocation or partial dislocation (sublaxation). This involves the ball of your lower jaw slipping out of the socket in your upper jaw, preventing you from closing your mouth and giving rise to the commonly used term "locked jaw." This generally only happens if you twist it suddenly, during an accident, for example, or while yawning. A doctor can manipulate a dislocated jaw back into the correct position using the so-called Hippocratic method. This is painful but not really dangerous and the sooner it happens, the fewer complications you have to worry about. Nevertheless, your jaw may need to be stabilized for a while afterwards.

One more thing: If you lock your jaw, you'll know it. There is no way you can confuse it with a slight hyperextension or sprain. If you can feel your jaw cracking or popping when you open your mouth too wide or for too long, it's nowhere near the same thing as dislocating it. That doesn't mean you shouldn't stop or be a bit more careful. There's no need to invite trouble.

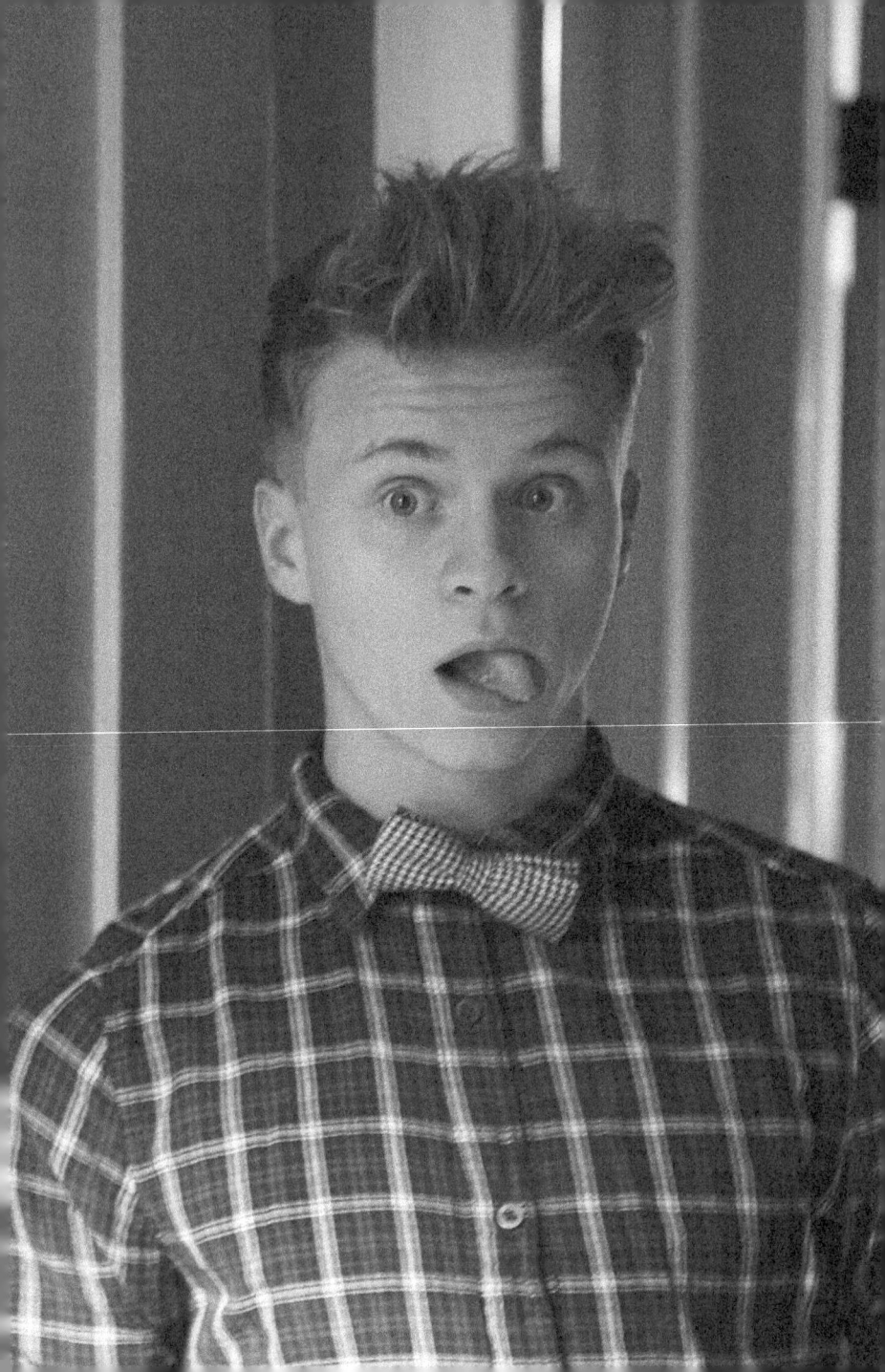

A Sore Tongue
This isn't really an injury, but if it crops up in unexpected places, you might think it is. If you use your tongue extensively when giving your partner a blow job, or spend an epic amount of time rimming him without any kind of prior training, don't be surprised if your tongue hurts slightly the next day whenever you move it. This will generally pass quickly and you'll be ready for the next session in no time at all. Regular licking sessions or practice sessions on your own in front of the mirror will provide a long-term solution to this problem.

INJURY RISKS FOR BOTTOMS

Dickless!
If you really want to cause a paranoia and masculinity-anxiety induced stampede, just shout the word "castration" and you're guaranteed to get the attention of just about every male on the planet. The "penis bitten off during oral sex" is a set piece in oodles and oodles of crime or horror fiction (see for example Felice Picano's *The Lure*). But let's get real here: The people seriously posting question such as "Are glory holes dangerous?" in Internet forums are all really just screwed-up heterosexuals worried about those "gay perverts" attacking their manhood. So let's be realistic: If bite attacks do happen, they always happen in the context of either self-defense or psychopathy. Besides, nobody has ever had his dick bitten clean off, because that would simply take a long time and extreme dedication to do. So you can uncross your legs now.

Ruptured Testicles and Co.
Sucking balls is a nice addition to your blow job repertoire and one that I can unreservedly recommend. But it does require a certain amount of skill on the part of the top. Ball sacks and their contents vary just as much if not more than dicks do with regard to consistency and sensitivity. So it's not entirely impossible or even improbable for a top to be slightly careless when handling

his partner's scrotum and hurting him by for example pulling his balls down too abruptly. Despite this, the fear of tearing off one or even both testicles that many have endured in this kind of scenario is in most cases entirely baseless. It takes a lot of rough handling, rougher than a during a clumsily given blow job, to rupture, bruise or otherwise cause trauma to your testicles. Likewise, testicular torsion (twisting the spermatic cord and cutting off the blood supply to the testicle) is generally not caused by sexual activity. This doesn't happen anyway unless your testicles are hypermobile, which is itself a relatively rare condition.

But now I've sounded the all-clear signal, that's no excuse for carelessness. If sucking your balls is painful, you won't get a special manliness cookie for continuing. Take a break and see what happens. In most cases, the pain will ease up quickly and you'll be back in business. If the pain persists, or if you experience nausea, swelling or redness around your scrotum, go straight to the emergency room or consult your urologist. You may need surgery to fix it.

Bruising/Burst Blood Vessels
Your penis is chock full of blood vessels. Otherwise it wouldn't get hard. However, wherever there's a vein or an artery, there's always the risk of it being damaged. This leads to hematomas, otherwise known as bruising. Yes, you can bruise your dick. So if your partner grips or bites your wang too hard (during oral sex, for example), you may end up with a black eye somewhere other than your face. A lot of times this goes unnoticed until later when you're in the shower. Sometimes it is only visible once your dick is fully erect. If you don't feel pain or any other symptoms, it is generally harmless and will go away after a couple of days. But if it gets worse, see a doctor!

Contusions and Fractures
Many men live in fear of breaking their penis. Which is why whenever stories of penile fractures hit the media, there is an uproar of panicky chattering among the male population. But in reality, these

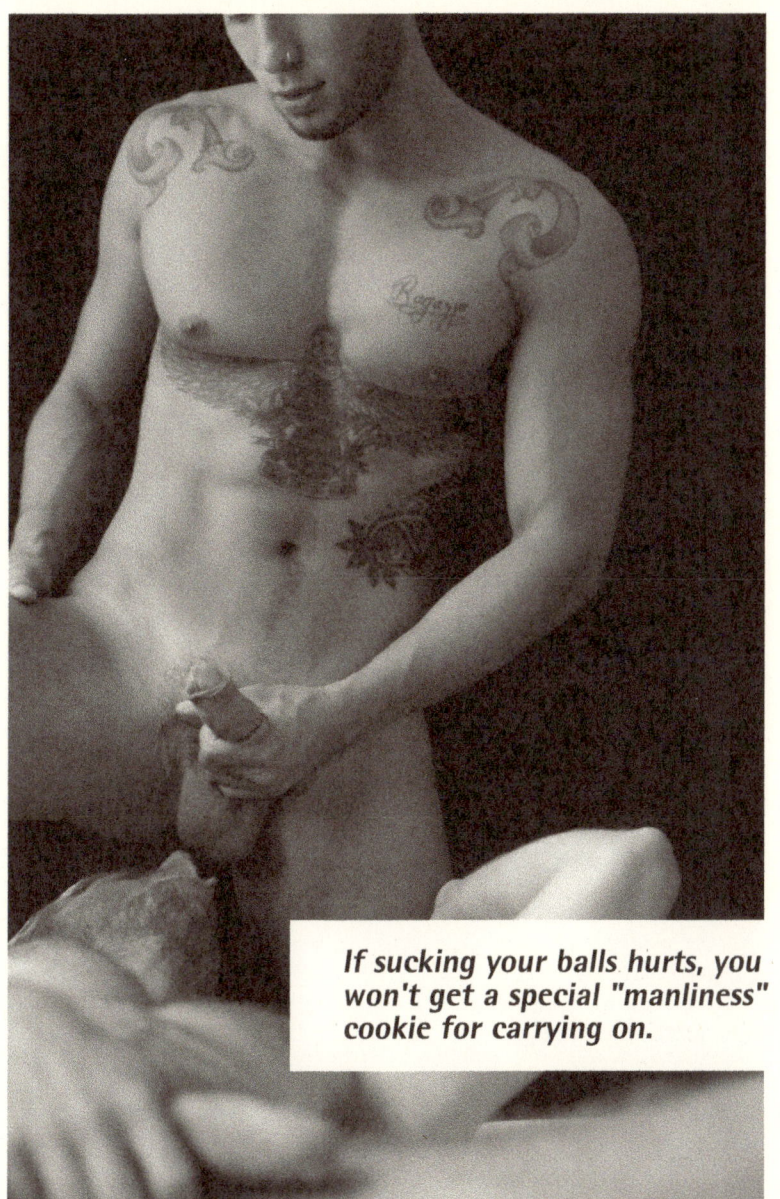

If sucking your balls hurts, you won't get a special "manliness" cookie for carrying on.

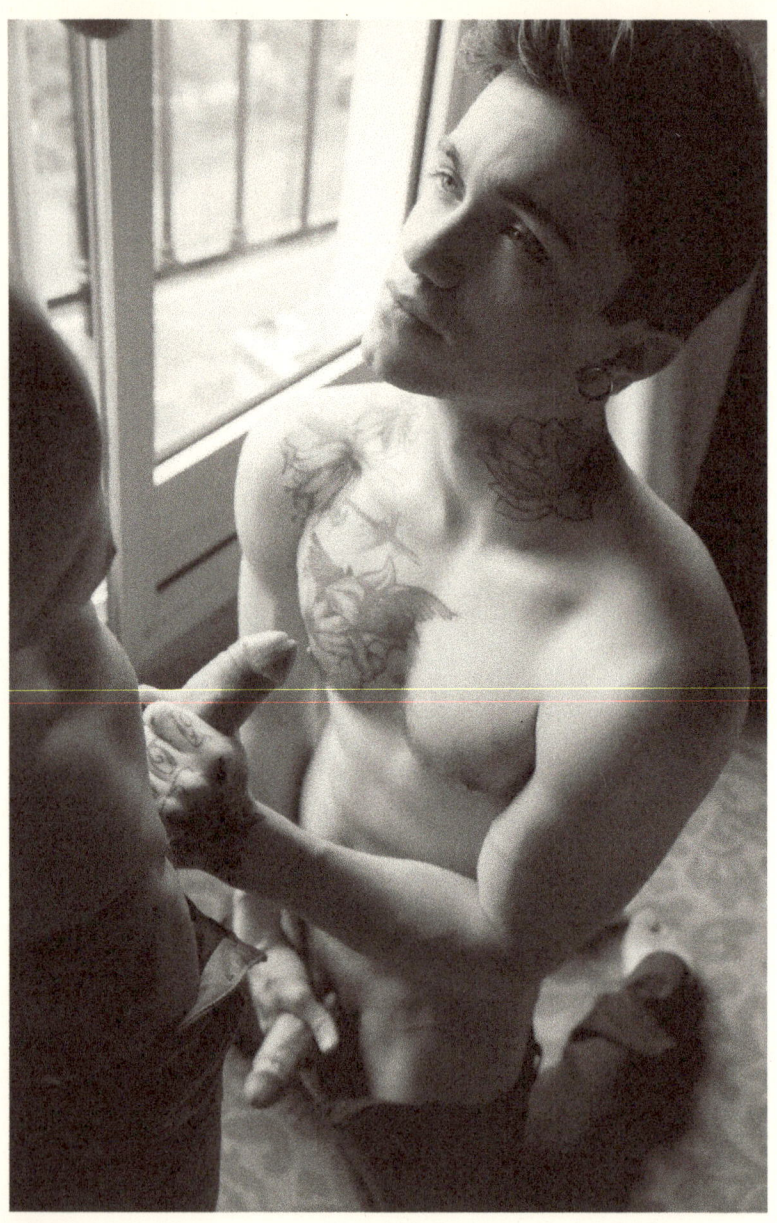

cases are extremely rare and highly unlikely. At least, as long as the top doesn't deliberately and maliciously twist or bend his partner's boner. Or to quote Hamburg urologist Christian Aust, who was featured in *The Bigger Bang*, "The penis consists of three so-called cavernous bodies of erectile tissue—one on each side and one, the corpus spongiosum, around the urethra. These bodies are made of sponge-like, are enveloped in a case of relatively hard skin. If this skin is torn due to one of the causes mentioned above, this results in blood leaking out of the cavernous bodies. Depending on how large the tear is, your penis will look like an uncooked sausage—large, blue, and floppy. If this happens, you should go straight to hospital, where the tear will be sewn up again. But as I said, this is a very rare occurrence."

> *Whenever stories of penile fractures hit the media, there is an uproar of panicky chatter among the male population.*

▼ Why does giving someone a blow job make your mouth water?

Human saliva performs the following functions: it keeps your mouth clean, washes away bacteria, and is an aid to digestion. As its production is governed by the autonomic nervous system, smelling or even just seeing tasty food can be enough to get your juices flowing. It's your body preparing for digestion. Does a nice juicy dick have the same effect as tasty food? Not really. Instead, increased saliva production during oral sex can be explained by the stimulation of the oral cavity, similar to when you're eating or chewing.

Theory Exam: Which Blow Job Department Is the Best Fit for You?

1: The phrase "Open wide!" makes you think of...

... being at the dentist.

... how to say it authoritatively.

I'm not here to think. I'm here to obey.

2: Spit on a dick smells...

... incredibly hot.

... takes some getting used to.

Huh? What am I supposed to be smelling here?

3: When you're jerking off, you generally use...

... just my hand and my imagination, or porn.

... spit or lube for added slipperiness.

I'd rather save my spunk for my next date.

4: The term "cock gobbler" is...

... a compliment.

... misleading. Not all of them are actually any good at oral.

A pick-up line that's guaranteed to fail!

5: Your views on masturbators:

If you're that desperate!

Sure. Better not run out of lube!

I wouldn't mind trying one out.

6: "Facials" are ...

... fine, as long as I'm the one giving them.

... an integral part of sex. I love them.

... an unacceptable expression of contempt.

7: Visit a glory hole and we'll see you ...

... on my knees with my mouth open.

... with my boner in the hole, hoping someone bites.

... elsewhere. Blow jobs without any eye contact don't do it for me.

8: Which statement do you agree with the most?

Oral sex without fucking is like porn with no dicks.

If you like dick, you'll love blow jobs.

The best blow job is a long blow job.

Your score: *Have you checked all the answers? Then let's take a look at your score. This is how it works: You'll find a different animal after each answer. The animals pictured here are either LAND, AIR, or WATER dwellers. Just count which element you've checked the most and then turn to the respective category on the following pages and find out, what that says about you.*

▼ Land Animals

Normally, if anyone asked if you were a blow job bottom, you would say yes—if you weren't so allergic to the term "bottom." Because you're a top, aren't you, you stud? In any case, you appear to have forged a very close relationship with your own dick over the course of your genital socialization and your main objective is to stick it into as many orifices as possible. You're not terribly picky about where, but you are quite impatient. You do not suffer inexperienced wannabe blow job artists gladly. And that's the crux of the matter. I don't have to tell you that there are any amount of inexperienced tops out there, but maybe I should point out that you can't insist on a deep-throat job from a beginner. Show a little indulgence to clumsy tops and use your own endurance to open their eyes and mouths. This will frequently be worth the effort in the long run. And let me ask you this question: Do you think your own experience in giving blow jobs might be a little limited? If you want to gain a better understanding of your partner's mistakes, it can't hurt to switch sides once in a while—even if it's just for the purposes of research. Hone your other skills by reading the chapter "Shut Your Eyes!" on page 108.

▼ Water Animals

You have a very sober relationship with your own sexuality. This has its advantages, especially as it stops you from doing anything risky. On the other hand, it does make you a bit of a snob. The combination of not-wanting-to-learn-from-others and not-being-especially-inventive is a sexual dead end. Think about it. Have you thought about it? And you're not offended? Good, you're not that much of a snob after all. Maybe you don't have much of an affinity to blow jobs simply because you've never had one? Or because they've never been terribly exciting? Or because you'd just rather fuck? There are many possible reasons but the real question is whether any of them prevents you from engaging with the subject of oral sex in the first place. If that's the case, then there is nothing I can do. On the other hand, you are currently reading a book called *The Better Blow Job*. This does at least suggest that you might have the will to discover new realms of pleasure. Whether it's as a top or a bottom is a question you might want to decide spontaneously, or you could look at your answers to see which signs you've checked the most, apart from the WATER animals. If you're a LAND animal, turn to page 108. AIR dwellers, just turn the page.

▼ Air Animals

You are actually overqualified for this book. If your hunger for cocks is as great as your answers would suggest, no one can teach you anything about sucking dick that you don't know already. However ... greed is not the same thing as enjoyment, and a big mouth does not always guarantee top quality. So don't let your unbridled greed for dicks stop you from sparing a thought for the guys attached to those dicks. It can't hurt to give them and yourself a break now and then. As long as you're not on the receiving end of a bukkake orgy, there's no harm in taking things slow. And if you are, you might want to take a few days off afterwards to process your experience. This will stop you from becoming too driven and washed out. Those AIR animals with a tendency towards addictive behavior should take this advice to heart. Everyone else can just be pleased with their oral talents and read the "Open Up" chapter on page 46, just to confirm how overqualified they actually are. After all, a little theory can't stop you from enjoying your practical experience. So, turn the page, please!

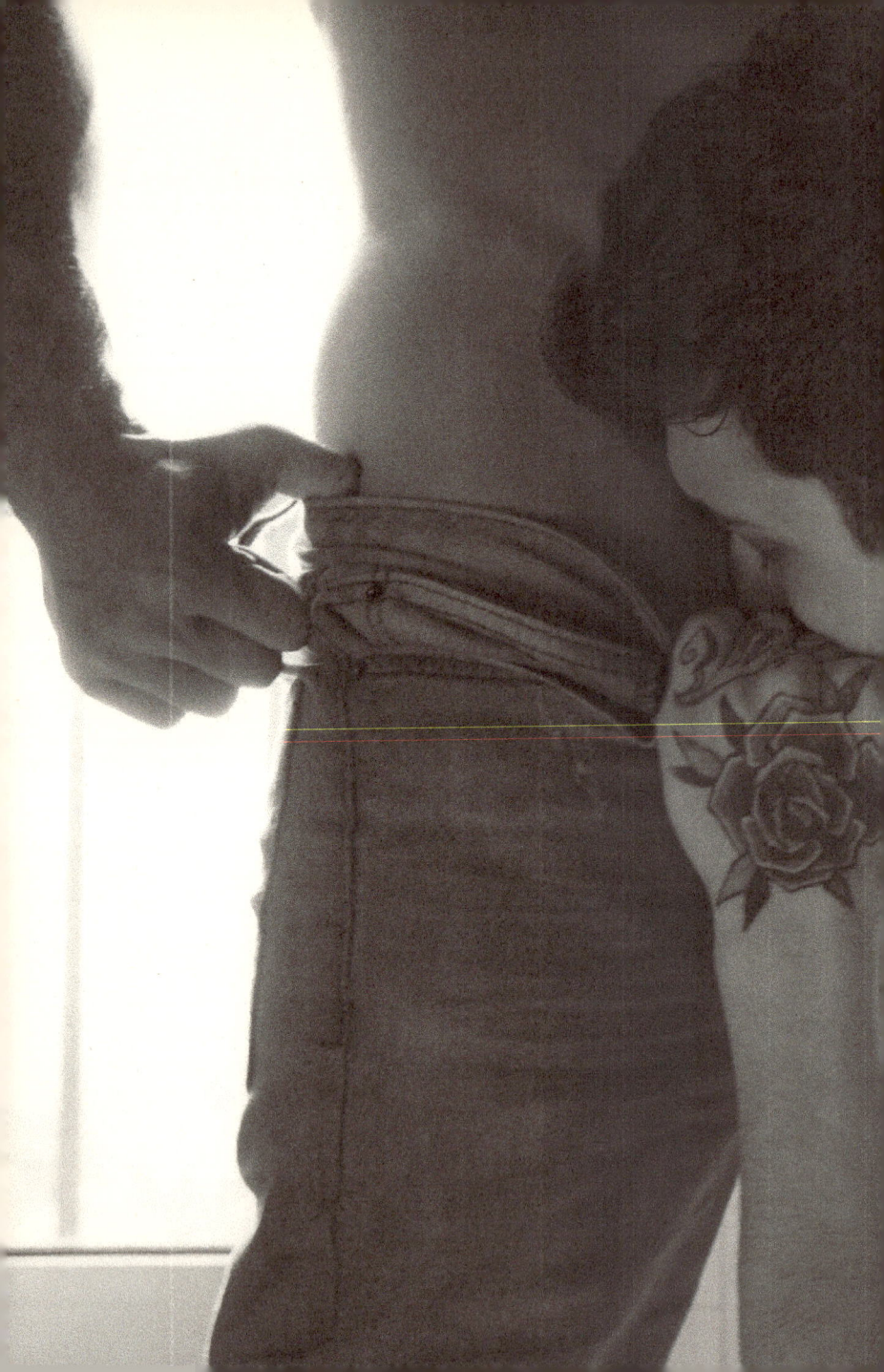

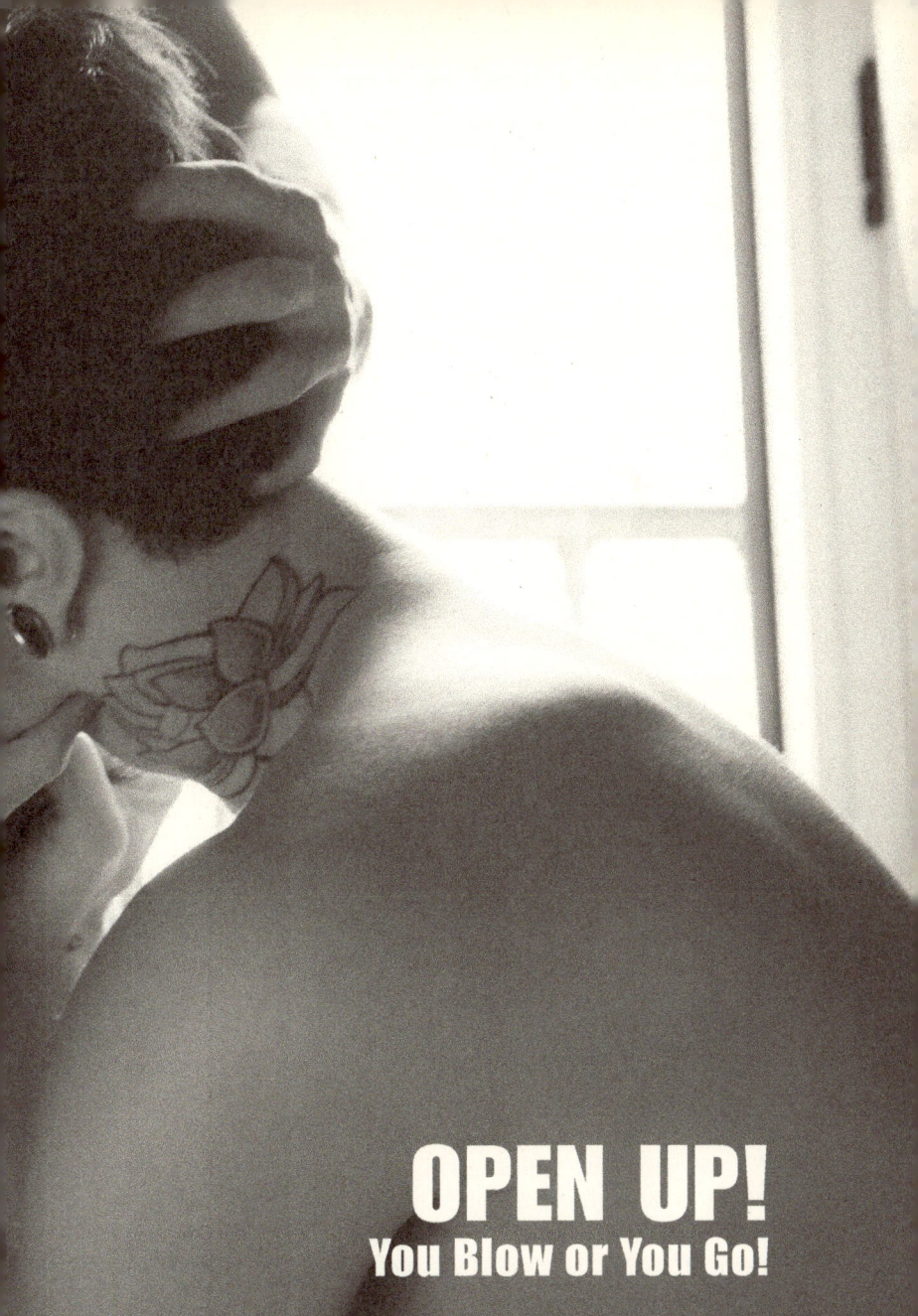

Open Up!

Basic Positions: Taking a Stand

Welcome to the dick worshippers' section! We're among friends here, so let's get comfortable and have a chat. The aim of this chapter is to help you identify, hone, or develop your personal skills. A lot of this will involve creating an awareness both of your own actions and your partner's needs. I've also thrown in a few practical exercises for which you will need some equipment, but I'll go into these later on.

First of all, I'd like to direct your attention to a pretty fundamental point. Anyone who has ever tried to give someone a blow job in a train restroom or on a ship at sea knows just how difficult and complicated sucking a dick on unsteady ground is. There is not much you can do about the circumstances, but they do serve to illustrate just how important a firm footing is for oral sex. The same applies on steady ground. So unless you want to turn every blow job into an exercise in agility, the following positions are best avoided.

The unsupported squat: This is hard work and will make your knees ache after a while. You also run the risk of being tipped backwards if your partner thrusts too hard.

The standing bend: Not relaxed and certainly not sexy! It is really difficult to get your mouth around your partner's dong at the right angle from this position. It also makes you look as if you're afraid of getting the knees of your pants dirty.

Flat on your back: Unless giving up all control is the entire point of the exercise, this position has little to recommend it. Any input on your part will be hell on your neck muscles. Apart from that, there are only two reasons you might want to opt for the supine position. First, for a 69 (although this is a lot more fun with both of you lying on your sides). Second, you want your partner to give your mouth a solid pounding from above. (Again, this is easier if you kneel down in front of the bottom with his hand steadying the back of your head.)

By contrast, I can always recommend any of the three basic positions.

On your knees: This has obvious advantages. It gives you a relatively firm grounding. It leaves both your hands free to direct your partner's cock, tickle his balls, or jerk him off. If your partner is standing up, his crotch will, in most cases, be at more or less the same level as your head. If he sits or lies down on the edge of the bed, you can kneel down between his legs and slobber away. So far, so good. Admittedly, there is the disadvantage of getting your pants dirty, especially if you're at an outdoor cruising spot, and it can be quite hard on your knees. If you're particularly sensitive to either of these things, put something under your knees first. Or wear kneepads. You may have trouble finding someone who thinks that's particularly sexy, though.

On all fours: Have your partner lie down flat on his back on the bed or the floor with his knees bent and crawl between his legs on all fours for great access. You can prop yourself up with your hands on his thighs and lower your open mouth over his boner, grab his hard-on in your fist and start licking, or switch to an impromptu 69 position—anything goes. It's a very stable position.

Sitting down: The alternative position for non-crawlers and those with tender knees! The great thing about this position is that it's incredibly comfortable and you can even support your back against the wall or the back of a chair. Other advantages will depend on how high your seat is. If you sit on a medium height stool with your back to the wall, your bottom can easily approach from the front and stick his junk in. The wall behind you provides great stability, especially if you're into deep-throating. If you only have a plain chair, you're going to have to lean forwards. Or you can have your bottom stand on a medium sized stool, but this doesn't provide him with much stability.

Whatever position you choose, the general rule is: anything goes. As long as you both enjoy it, and if you enjoy tying yourselves into knots, then go right ahead. But if this detracts from your enjoyment, you may want to return to the tried and true basic positions. Other factors generally work themselves out on their own, depending on your respective heights, differences in height, preferences and aversions, flexibility, and temperament. To find out more about the latter, why not try all of the aforementioned positions out in blow-job-simulation mode and then choose your favorite. If that isn't necessary, turn directly to page 53 to find out what your blow job type is. Or if you need a short break, you can go shopping instead. We're going to need a couple of utensils for the practical exercises later on, so it's a good idea to have them to hand. If you want to get really stuck in, take a good look at this shopping list—or you can tear it out or take a photo of it—and go on a quick shopping trip before you read on.

BETTER SHOPPING: A SHOPPING LIST FOR TOPS

- cucumber

- blindfold

- bananas

- popsicles

- handheld mirror

- condoms

- knife

- paper towels

- champagne glass

You can always use a (not too large) model phallus. If you don't own one, add the following to your list:

- dildo

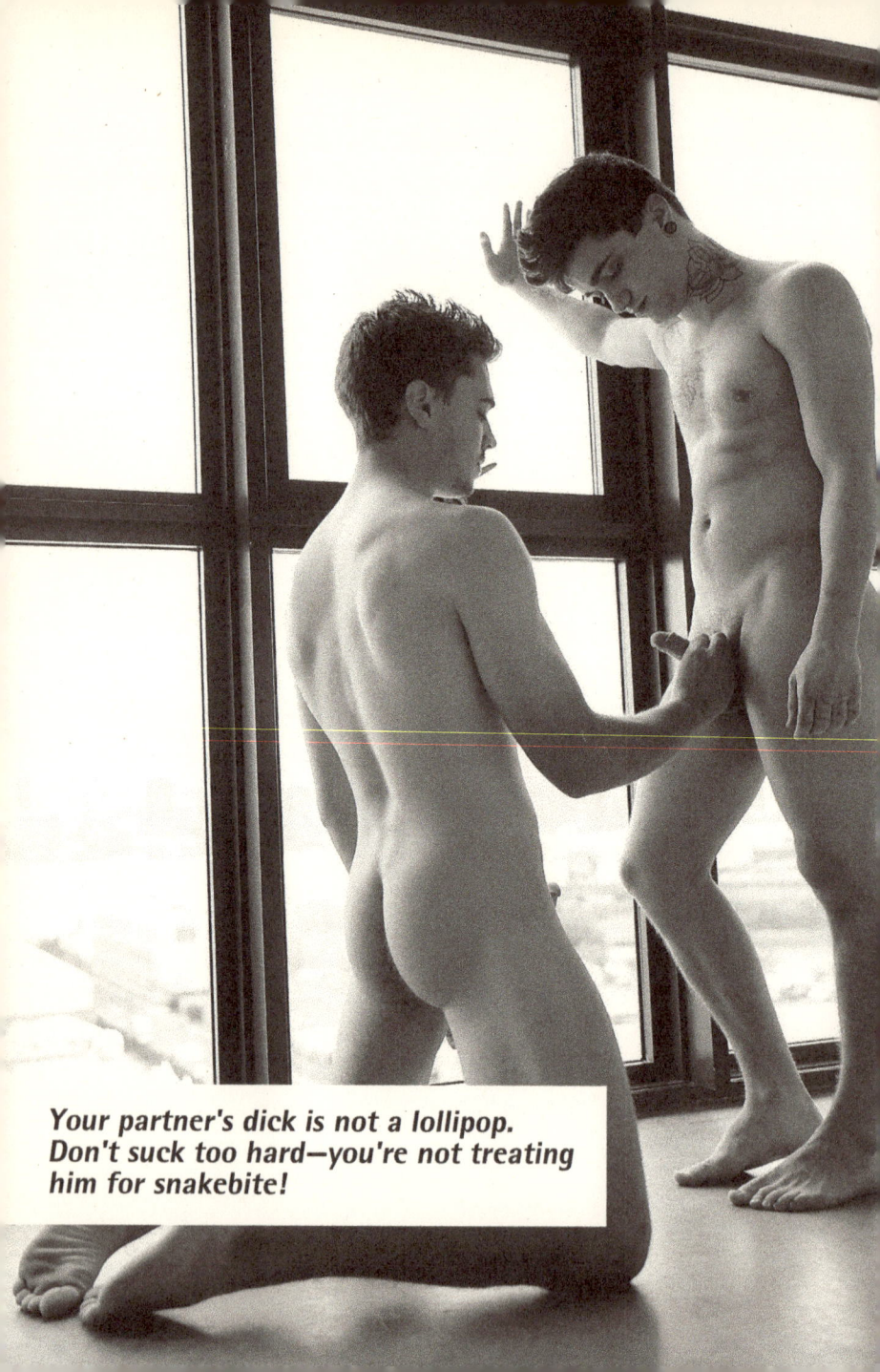

What's Your Blow Job Type?

Not everyone gives blow jobs the same way; most people have specialties they have developed over time. You know yourself what works intuitively and what doesn't work. But sometimes, this leads to a kind of playing-it-safe mentality, and you forget that there are other options. So the following list of blow job types is not only for you to identify your own style and the most compatible topping styles. It also aims at making you aware of other methods you may have been neglecting. Ideally, you should have every blow job type lying dormant inside of you, just waiting for the right moment (the right type of bottom) to call it into action.

▼ Suckers

It's not just the look of dicks that turns you on, you love the way they smell and taste as well? Then you're a sucker and part of the gourmet faction. There's no need for me to explain this term, but I will mention a couple of things you might want to keep an eye on when sucking cock. First of all, your partner's dick is not a lollipop. There are very few bottoms out there who enjoy having their dick sucked as if you were trying to treat them for snakebite. So don't overdo it, and look up from time to time to make sure your efforts are actually being appreciated. The sensitivity of the glans varies from person to person (whether or not they are circumcised). So proceed with caution. On the other hand, you can also set a few stimulation points of your own. Again, eye contact can be helpful here. There's a very nice maneuver that I like to call "jerksucking," which is equally enjoyable for the top and the bottom. It involves sucking the tip of your partner's penis while stroking up and down the shaft. It's also great preparation for deep-throating!
Compatible with: pashas, Mr. Sensitive

▼ Fluffers

You don't beat around the bush (ha!); you're purposeful, ambitious and you know exactly how to get your partner in the mood? Then you, my friend, have earned the right to call yourself a "fluffer." Back in the golden age of porn, this term was used to refer to the unseen heroes of every porno movie. Their job was to stiffen up a tired pro's flagging equipment whenever needed. These days, most companies have replaced the human fluffer with chemical erection enhancers, usually to save costs. That doesn't matter. Because you can still find the same level of skill and motivation without a financial incentive. I don't really have much advice to give this group. A large part of their oral talent consists of being able to adapt their skills to their partners' needs. I would however like to point out just one thing: Gaining satisfaction from the knowledge of a job well done is great. But you should also show it from time to time. Most bottoms will appreciate if their tops vocalize freely or otherwise express their own personal satisfaction with what they are doing. Some fluffers tend to forget about this in the course of the dogged pursuit of their duties. Before your partner starts asking himself whether you're even having fun, you might want to ask yourself that question from time to time.
Compatible with: humpers, jizzers, fappers

▼ Gaggers

You're tough and untiring; you like to surrender yourself up to your partners and don't mind a bit of rough treatment now and then. Then you are probably already familiar with the magic word "gagging." In the context of oral sex, this refers to the exciting gurgling, spitting, and sniffing caused by intense deep-throat sessions. This is clearly a category for more advanced practitioners. Few people can shove an entire dick down their throats and enjoy it without a lot of practice.

> **Only more advanced practitioners are into gurgling and gagging.**

Which is why this book is also designed to help you learn the skill, step by step. Kudos if you've already gotten this far on your own. Enjoy! The latter in particular. Why do I say this? In my experience, many adepts at extreme deep-throating tend to hit a wall in their pursuit of new harder-deeper-further kicks at some point. They then turn to quantity and drugs to compensate for the lack of new sexual challenges and thrills. The result is: gangbangs, BDSM, and druggy sex. There's nothing wrong with any of this in principle, as long as you're responsible and think about what you're doing. But some gaggers neglect both of these aspects. And that leads to them neglecting their own pleasure. It can't hurt to occasionally tell yourself that every new boner presents a new challenge. Even if it happens to be smaller than the last.

> *Every new boner presents a new challenge. Even if it happens to be smaller than the last.*

Compatible with: humpers, explorers

▼ Swallowers

As soon as you saw that this book had its own chapter on "Swallowing," were you tempted to just skip ahead to the end? And the idea of millions of men jerking off on their own and emptying out their precious semen into urinals and socks seems like a terrible waste? Then you're probably a passionate swallower. This category nearly became extinct in the wake of the AIDS crisis, but it has since been steadily on the increase. Besides the blow job itself, the main erotic thrill here is swallowing cum. I have already stated that this is not a safe practice and any other points will be cleared up in full in the "Swallowing" chapter, which I strongly recommend for anyone who conforms to this blow job type. Apart from that, most swallowing aficionados are just as obsessed with dicks as they are with semen, which means that are frequently just as talented as all the fluffers and gaggers out there. In those rare cases where giving a blow job has been downgraded to being a necessary precursor to milking your partner, I can only advise the swallower, in his interest, to do a solid job. In any case, it is always helpful to communicate your special interest beforehand. This also applies to darkrooms. Surprise blow jobs, where you abruptly increase the tempo, momentum, and depth as soon as you notice that the other guy is well on the road to orgasm, may be an efficient way of getting what you want, but they are not really fair on the bottom.

Compatible with: jizzers, fappers, explorers

▼ Lickers

You are a great believer in the saying that the tongue is the strongest muscle in your body and you categorically reject the idea that all blow jobs should end up in a deep-throat session? You presumably know what you're talking about. Because you're a licker. Instead of adapting the old in-and-out to oral circumstances, you prefer to tickle your partner to orgasm with the skillful use of your tongue. You might say that this art form does not, strictly speaking, belong in the blow job category at all, but you might also call it the supreme discipline. It takes a lot of virtuosity to keep the boners of the world standing to attention with just your tongue. Which leads us to the crux of the matter: The guild of lickers is not a haven for those who simply can't or won't get their mouths around their partners' dicks. Instead, it unites those men who, despite having a mouth full of cock, are able to stretch their tongues out, past their lower lips, and use them to caress the underside of the shaft. I have the greatest respect for these men. They should however always remember that there are some bottoms out there who are entirely content with a bit of oral in-and-out, but simply can't deal with intense lingual play. So don't turn your nose up at the coarser options.

Compatible with: pashas, Mr. Sensitive

▼ Biters

You like nothing more than gently nibbling your partner's semi-chub through the fabric of his underpants? When the pants come down, you like to massage his shaft with your teeth? Or bite his foreskin and tug it gently? Then you're either a dangerous lunatic or a real pro. Using your teeth during a blow job is tricky and not to be undertaken lightly. For one thing, there is a distinct risk of injuring your partner and for another, some bottoms find it really unpleasant. The somewhat brutal term "biter" doesn't really do justice to the true representatives of this type. Aside from a penchant for using their teeth, they are characterized by a high degree of skill and sensitivity. Because they know that the soft skin of your dick is still sensitive, even when it's hard. However, the fun stops as soon as you get a broken tooth, or any other sharp or jagged edges. If that happens, place your skills in the service of any one of the abovementioned categories until your dentist has fixed you up again.
Compatible with: pashas, explorers

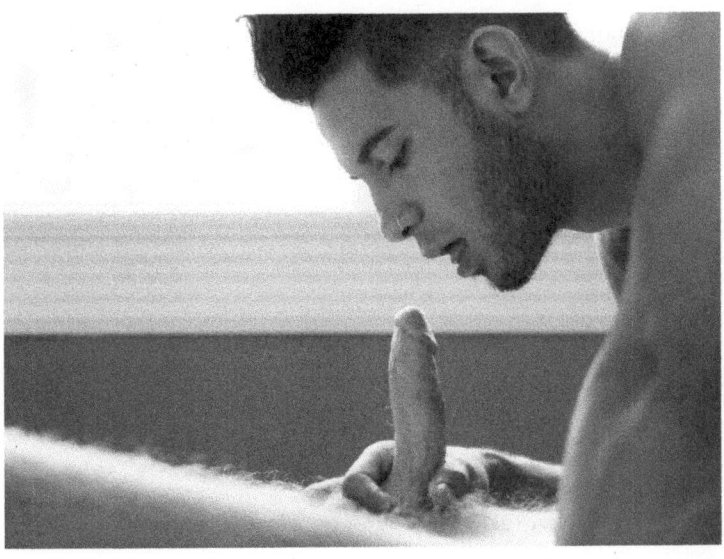

A Blow Job Artist's Basic Equipment

The blow job types described above emphasize or even represent the individual body parts employed during a blow job: Lickers represent the tongue, suckers represent the oral cavity, gaggers represent the throat, and biters represent the teeth. But that doesn't answer the question of how to employ these individual body parts to best effect. This is the subject of the following section. It also includes a couple of other "utensils" you should definitely avail yourself of when giving a blow job. First and foremost: your hands. Which is why we're going to start with them.

▼ Hands

No, your hands are not just for playing with your own boner while you're giving your partner a blow job. They are also a major factor in making oral sex an even more intense experience for both of you. As long as you use them properly. Here's a selection of ways you can use your hands.

The ball noose: Using your index finger and thumb, make a loop around the top of your partner's scrotum and then tug down gently (or more firmly, if you both want to); it's a surefire guarantee for moans of pleasure from above.

Fist: This blow job all-rounder grip can be employed in a variety of ways. First of all, you can use it to give yourself a break. Wrap your fist around your partner's boner and give it a couple of vigorous faps to keep stimulation levels up while you take a quick breather.

The cuff: A classic move for especially well-endowed partners. Wrap your fist around the root of the bottom's penis and just leave it there while you blow him. This not only has the advantage of allowing you to enhance his erection with a couple of pumping movements, it also "shortens" his boner by those couple of inches that might otherwise be too much for your throat.

Another popular move and especially appealing for uncut partners: Take the glans into your mouth and suck while at the same time slowly (at first—you can increase the pace gradually) jerking off the shaft.

A sensitive touch: Speaking of foreskins ... if your partner has one, you should definitely not neglect it. As everybody knows, the stronger the erection, the more difficult it is to suck while sticking your tongue into the opening, because the foreskin generally slides back behind the glans. And that's where a sensitive touch can help you. If you push the skin of your partner's shaft forwards with your fist and then grab the foreskin cap with the tips of the fingers on your other hand, you can pull it apart. Now let your tongue circle around the tip inside the opening to produce an incredibly hot sensation for yourself and sensual fireworks for your partner. It can even be a little too much for some people, but

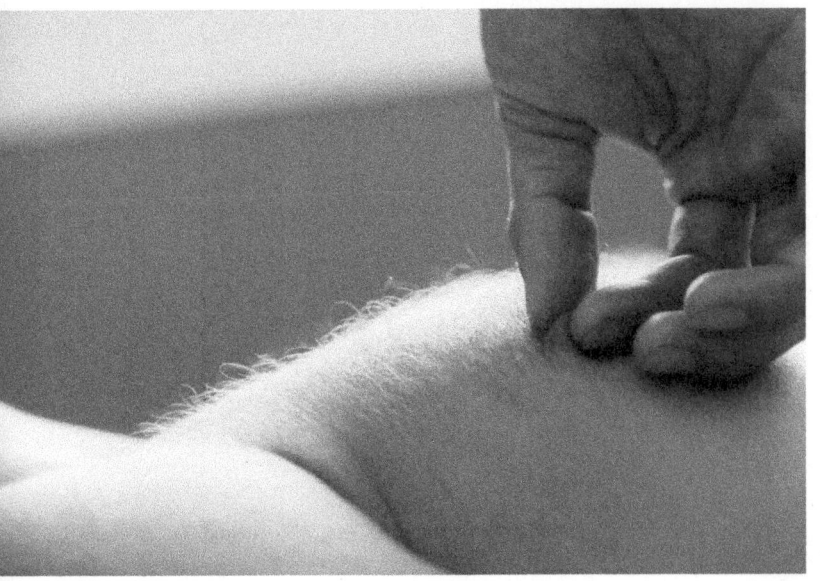

you'll notice if that's the case. Besides this special and especially hot scenario, you can also use your fingertips to add extra sensation pretty much everywhere. You can slide them up and down both sides of his groin. You can carefully touch his spit-lubed boner while you take a quick break. You can reach up and shove them in your partner's mouth. You can massage his nipples—or his testicles (which is also a great way to occupy your free hand when you're performing the ball noose). You can keep that up for a while. The only limits to your creativity are generally a lack of multitasking skills. Your motor skills may not be at their best while you're giving enthusiastic head.

> **The only limits to your creativity are generally a lack of multitasking skills.**

Ass vise and hip clamp: Your hands can play an invaluable part in regulating the vigor of a blow job. They can be used to both intensify and soften the impact. A hip clamp involves you holding your thrust-happy lover's thigh in both hands to tame his madly plunging hips. Ass-clamping, on the other hand (grabbing hold of your partner's ass cheeks with both hands and pushing him forwards), can help you push your partner's dick in and out of your mouth with as much force and depth as you like.

▼ Eyes

What do people always say about gourmet cooking? "A feast for the eyes as well?" This applies just as much to oral sex. Most arousal takes place in your brain. Hormones, smell, and touch all play a part, but so does sight. Which is why your eyes also play a role during oral sex. There is nothing hotter than an enthusiastic blow job artist gazing up into his partner's eyes while swallowing his sword. Conversely, there is nothing more boring and inhibiting than a top toiling away in his partner's lap without even once looking up. So let your eyes do the talking, you guys. It's like watching porn for your partners. And they also communicate loads of information, whether you want it or not: Do you enjoy the taste of his dick? Do you want more? Are you having fun? Can't you get enough of it? Of course, the answer your top wants to each of these questions is "yes." As talking with your mouth full just isn't polite, you can use your eyes to get the message across. Apart from the fact that being literally "looked up to" will give your partner an ego boost which will hopefully communicate itself to his erection.

▼ Lips

To enter your mouth, every dick is going to have to get past your lips. The only question is whether or not it can feel them. We will go into a couple of excellent deep-throat variations that deliberately avoid touching the lips later on, but you can also use them to add extra sensation. The anatomical foundation of your lips consists of a muscular ring, the so-called musculus orbicularis oris. It is also known as the kissing muscle, as this is what enables us to pucker up our lips into a kiss.

> *The musculus orbicularis oris is also known as the kissing muscle.*

There's a whole spectrum of options in between clenching and relaxing. You can make snapping movements to massage the shaft. You can gradually increase the pressure while thrusting back and forth. You can push out your lower lip and rub it against the glans. Or you can swallow his boner up to the hilt and squeeze your lips around the root of his penis. With a little practice, you can achieve a kind of cock ring effect, which will make his hard-on feel like it's swelling up inside your mouth. The muscles around your mouth can be trained, as illustrated by the "lip bodybuilding" training undertaken by many trombone and trumpet players to increase both the strength and the coordination of the muscles used for playing the trumpet. Special barbells and expanders have been designed for this very purpose. The former consist of a bar with tiny weights suspended from either end. These are "lifted" by holding the bar between your lips and keeping it there as long as you can. Expanders work according to a similar principle. Except that in this case, you don't build up lip strength using weights, but by holding onto a mouthpiece and gradually increasing the resistance by extending the expander bar. In my opinion, these measures are not necessary for a decent oral dick-massage, but if your lover wants more lip pressure on his dick, you might want to consider it.

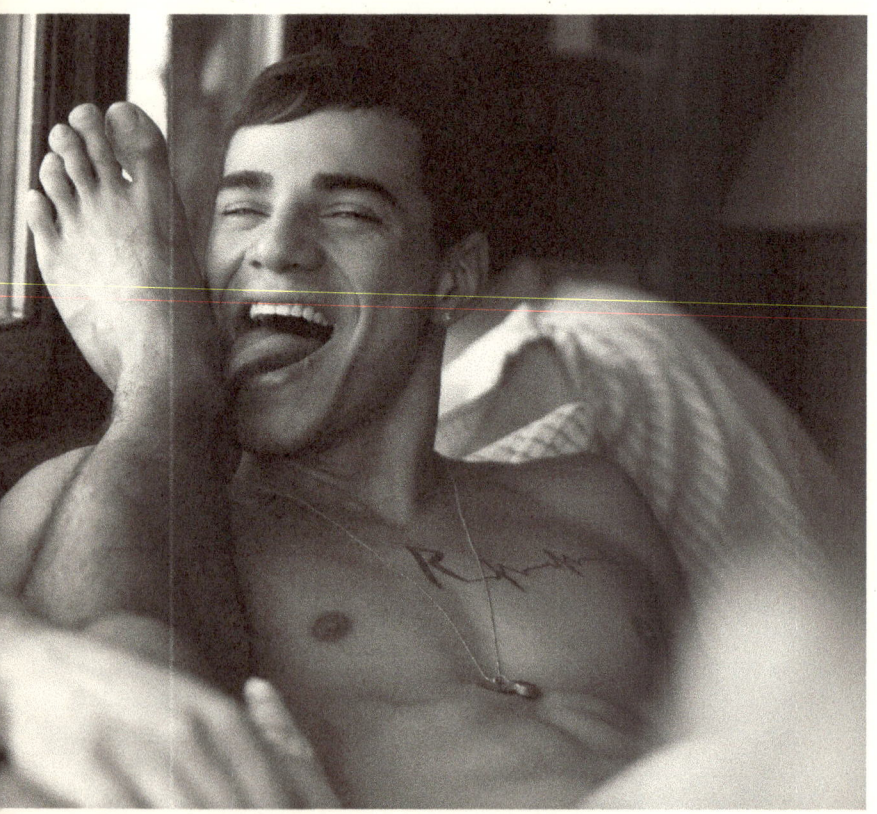

▼ Tongue

The muscles of your tongue are similar to those of your lips. They contribute a lot to the variety of a blow job and you can also train them. Three examples: Place a grape on your tongue and carefully stick it out and pull it back in again without dropping it to enhance your concentration. Stick one finger inside your mouth and push against it with your tongue (as if you were bench-pressing) to increase your strength. Stick your tongue out as far as it will go and keep it there for as long as you can, or pull it back as far as possible to increase your flexibility. But why would you want to do that? For longer and better kissing, for example. Or to help you pronounce unfamiliar sounds when you're learning a foreign language. Or, to use your tongue to give your blow jobs a certain je ne sais quoi. Apart from the special massage I described earlier in the section on "lickers," there are plenty of other possibilities. Here's a selection of the top three variations to whet your appetite.

The vertical washcloth: Lick your partner's boner clean until it gets dirty? You will need plenty of endurance or an incredibly sensitive partner, but the vertical washcloth is also a great warm-up technique. Once your partner's dick is nice and hard, push it up against his stomach and run your tongue slowly up the entire shaft in broad strokes, from his balls to the tip. Repeat a couple of times while increasing the pressure.

The glans propellor: Pull your partner's foreskin (if he has one) back behind the glans, stick your tongue out and carefully lick around the tip with a circular motion. If the glans has a strongly accentuated corona (ridge), you can also dab your tongue across the groove between the glans and the foreskin. Try it; it's great. At least, as long as your partner is clean, but you'll notice soon enough if anything smells funky. Please note: Not all bottoms will enjoy the glans propellor. If your partner is very sensitive and your oral skills make him wince, there is no point in carrying on.

The trampoline: Get down on your knees, sit up like a doggy, and stick out your tongue. Then tell your partner to tap your tongue with the tip of his penis. Or—to stick with the image—to jump on your trampoline. This variation is a popular element of puppy play. You can really get each other going this way, especially if it involves playing with dominance and submission. Of course, you both know that you're going to snap and attack him at some point.

▼ Voice

While using your eyes to create a visual real life porn feeling, you can also use your voice to do the same thing acoustically. I don't just mean the sounds you produce as a matter of course, I mean every kind of sound you can make during sex—moaning, hissing, panting, or dirty talk. The fact that you've got your mouth full, preventing you from actually speaking, shouldn't stop you from expressing your enjoyment in other ways. On the contrary. This communicates your own sensations to your partner and will increase his arousal. The involuntary gagging or gurgling, a by-product of merciless deep-throating sessions, are characteristic of the potential of sounds to arouse. These are physical reactions produced involuntarily—that is to say, authentically—as a result of sexual activity. I am aware that not everyone finds them pleasant in this case, but that isn't the point. The point is that gagging sounds and is completely authentic. The same principle should be applied to every vocal expression. What I'm trying to say is: You can go ahead and exaggerate your pants and moans, your "Yes, fuck my mouth!" if you like, but they should always be an extension of an actual sensation. That's what makes them hot. Prefabricated porn-track moaning always sounds forced, which generally isn't sexy. But for that matter, neither is total silence, as if you were brooding over a math test. To hit the sweet spot in between, you will have to find your own voice—a combination of awareness, relaxation, and just letting yourself go.

▼ Face

Sure, your lips, your eyes, your tongue—these are all parts of your face. But their special blow job functions warrant individual consideration. We should also take a look at the face in its entirety, however, as in the heat of the moment it is easy to forget its potential as a playing field. You get right down to sucking, licking, slurping, and swallowing, and all the time you've almost forgotten the essence, the driving force behind oral sex: dick worship. I know, that always sounds so religious and over the top. But now we're back to the face, why don't we try and give the term a more tender meaning? After all: If you like giving blow jobs, it's generally because you like dicks. Oral sex is a very active and consuming expression of this preference. For a sensual, perhaps even meditative addition, try rubbing the object of your desire with your nose, your cheeks or forehead. Give his boner a cuddle with your face. Of course, I use the term cuddle in the widest possible sense. Your range of "cuddling" techniques might also include consensual dick-slaps on either cheek. Or playfully pressing the tip of his cock against your eyelids (close your eyes first!). Or greedily sucking in the scent of his penis with your nose. In any event, your face provides a wealth of possibilities for adding a little spice to your worship, besides the oral attraction. Even if it's just to find out how your partner's dick responds to a rendezvous with your stubble.

Blow Job Boot Camp for Tops

"Atteeeen-shun!" Mouths open! Aaaand ... companeeeee blow!"

This kind of basic training camp is presumably a feature of many a man's wet dream—as long as it involves real dicks. There are gay kink and outdoor clubs that have set out to fulfill these fantasies—first and foremost the Green Berets, who are active around the world. Those who start to revel in fantasies of hardcore action the moment they hear the word "boot camp," can safely apply there. Everyone else can continue reading this rather silly, but instructive series of exercises designed to whet your appetite for deep-throating. (After all, that's what most blow job tops aspire to.) Those who would like to participate should have all the utensils listed on our shopping list on page 51 to hand. When choosing your champagne glass, make sure it's a tulip glass (flutes are unsuitable for our purposes). The cucumbers and bananas should be stored at room temperature, if possible, not refrigerated. The popsicles, on the other hand, should be taken straight from the deep freeze and not thawed out beforehand.

Before you head to the freezer, just a couple of words in advance: I freely confess I used to laugh long and hard at those advice sections in women's magazines telling their readers to use dildos, carrots, zucchini, and other veggies to prepare themselves for a blow job. In my opinion, these aids had only one purpose: Once you'd finished practicing with them, you were in a position to fully appreciate the flexibility of a real life dick. I was firmly convinced that you could only practice giving head properly with the real thing. My friends and I used to argue whether you would have to spend a couple of nights in front of a glory hole down at your trusted local porn theater in order to master the art of oral sex. In my opinion, yes, you did. Perhaps because that was the strategy I followed before I came out. I can also state that if you want a crash course in awareness for the variety of erectile angles, shapes and sizes, this method (which can of course also be practiced in cruising areas and darkrooms) is definitely instructive. And the fact that these situations frequently lead to your partner

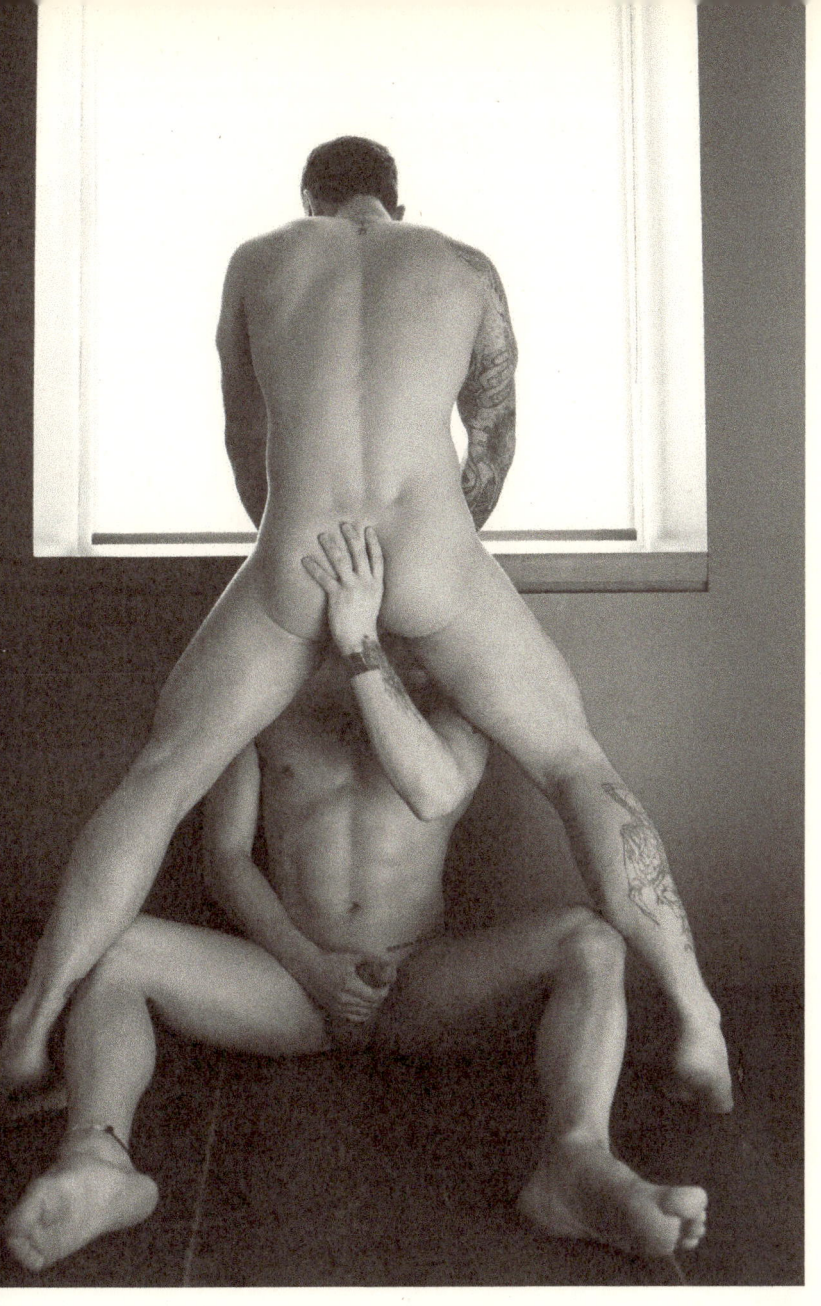

withdrawing his trust and his dick if you don't treat it well also teaches you a lot about how not to do it. But I am no longer convinced that this method is really the best for everyone. There are three reasons for this. First of all, I have since accepted that not everyone is comfortable in a darkroom or an adult movie theater, or even has access to one close by. Secondly, this strategy is so irresponsible and unsafe, there is no way I would feel right about recommending it to the general public. Thirdly, I took another, less arrogant and more lighthearted, look at the veggie option— and realized that, despite all its staid awkwardness, it did have its good points. What follows are three reasons I changed my mind. One: You can experiment with giving blow jobs to vegetables in the safety of your own home, without the pressure of having anyone else around. Two: If you're preparing for a deep-throat blow job, it can be particularly helpful to practice with a replacement phallus instead of bungling the job with the original. Especially as you can easily hurt yourself if you're not careful. Three: If you try out the entire workout program as presented here, it can be an instructive and amusing ritual. You can perform it on your own, with your best buddy, or even your best girlfriend. And now, my dears, place all the items on your shopping list on a table in front of you! Then head straight to the freezer for a popsicle! We are going to need it for the first exercise.

▼ Exercise 1: Frozen Blow Job

Let's start out with this fun and tasty exercise! You'll need a popsicle and a bunch of paper towels to combat stains. Be prepared for a fair amount of dripping and dribbling. Apart from that, all you have to do is suck the tip of your popsicle until it's completely round and then push it as far back into your throat as possible. If you can find one, a popsicle with a long stick will have the advantage of providing you with an extra long phallus. But this is not really essential. The point of this exercise is not to completely fill your mouth, but rather to provoke the gag reflex in the back of your throat. Slowly push the popsicle down your throat until you think you can't go any further or until you start gagging. Try and keep it in that position for a couple of seconds and then pull it out again without breaking it. The last step can be quite a challenge and it generally only works if you avoid all contact with your lips and teeth and don't suck—which makes it a good method for helping you realize that a deep-throat blow job has nothing to do with sucking. The idea is rather to offer as little resistance as possible to enable you to keep the popsicle at the deepest point for as long as you can. The best way to do this is to hold your breath, as even breathing through your nose will constrict your throat. After that, how long you can keep it up and whether you can withstand any additional thrusting is largely a question of training. You can practice this with a frozen blow job as well. Once you have tried pushing it in, keeping it there, and pulling it out again a couple of times, you can extend the second stage by pushing the popsicle forwards and backwards in small thrusts. This will probably activate your gag reflex again. But that's your main objective. Taming the reflex entails being able to both assess and control it. Practicing with a popsicle isn't a bad idea. It tastes good, it melts after a while and the cold will combat the unfamiliar gag reflex. The rest is, as with every other exercise, a question of persistent repetition. So you will probably find yourself eating several popsicles. Don't make yourself sick!

> *Popsicles taste good; they melt, and the cold will help keep down your gag reflex.*

▼ Exercise 2: Seen Through a Glass

Now that we've become briefly acquainted with our gag reflex, we'll leave it alone for the duration of this exercise. Instead, we will take a look at three body parts that play a major part in oral sex: your tongue, teeth, and lips. You will need the champagne glass and a handheld mirror. First of all, pick up the glass. It should be clean, empty, and (as previously mentioned) tulip-shaped. Hold it up to your face, as if you were going to drink out of it, but then open your mouth wide and close your lips around the rim. If you have managed to do that, then push the glass carefully into your mouth. Careful! If it proves difficult, please stop immediately. Otherwise the risk of the glass breaking and injuring you is too great for you to let your pride and ambition push you to into biting off more than you can chew!

> *Looking through a glass, you will see there is a lot more space inside your mouth than you would expect.*

If you have however made it this far, you'll notice two things. First: You need to get it past your teeth. This means, be very, very careful! You don't want the glass to break, so you must stop yourself from biting down. This will prepare you for a hard dick, which is also fragile in its own way. Second: You will realize that by stretching the corners of your mouth, you can create a snapping movement with your lips, which will help you work the glass in. Your lips should inch their way down from the edge of the glass. You won't and shouldn't get very far, but this is a great method for learning how to work your way down a boner. Especially as you can now pick up your mirror and (if you have enough light) take a look inside your oral cavity through the glass. You will see that there is a lot more space than you would expect. Let me be very clear: The point is not to stuff the entire glass into your mouth but rather to use its shape and material to illustrate certain basic principles. So please, don't overdo it!

And now it's your tongue's turn! Most people will intuitively push their tongues down with the glass. This is the correct way to proceed. In some cases or situations, however, the superfluous tissue will be pushed inside the glass. Whichever way you proceed, your tongue will ultimately be responsible for preventing the glass from advancing any further. What does this tell us? Your tongue,

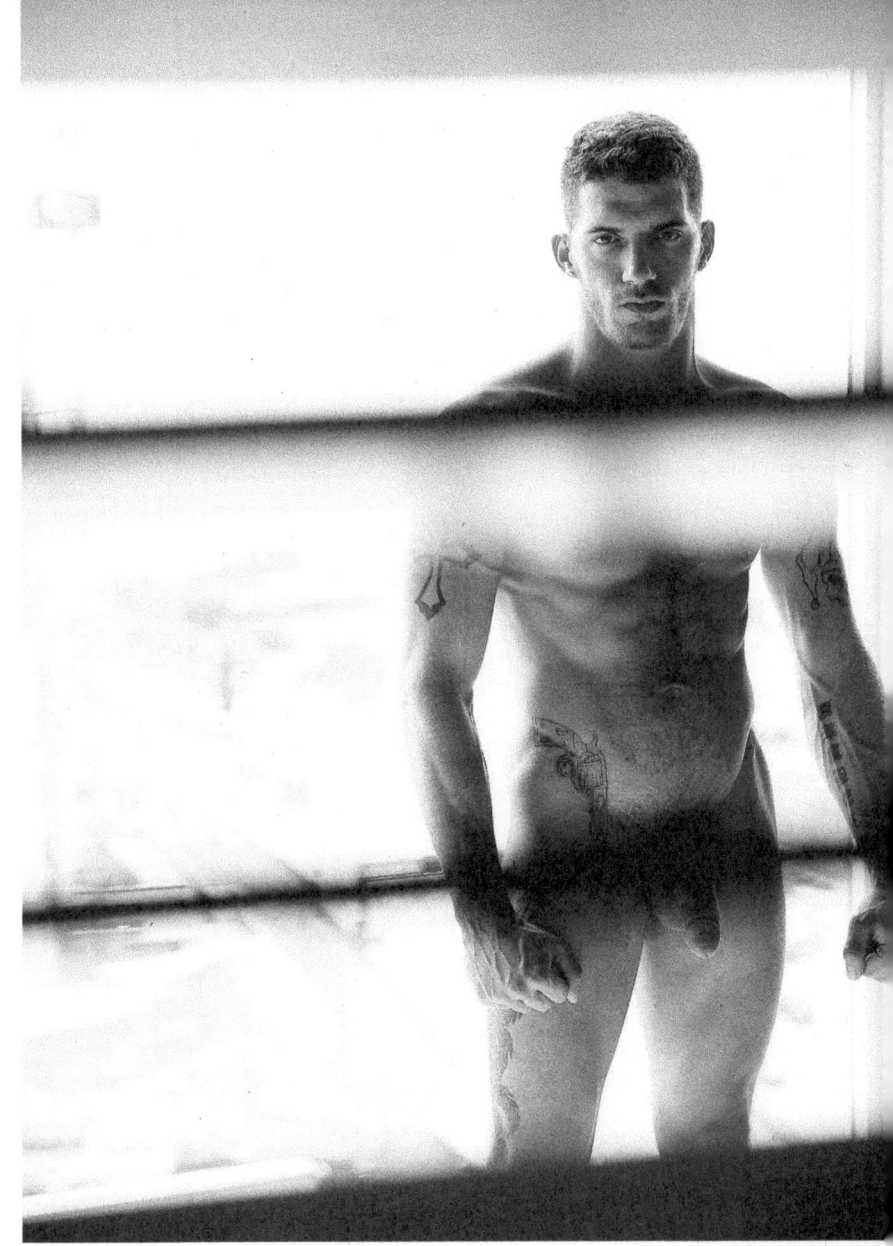

which plays the main role when you're licking someone's cock, will only get in the way during an actual blow job. So you will do yourself a big favor by keeping it as flat and still as possible. The "Seen Through a Glass" exercise can also provide us with further insights. For this, you will have to fill it halfway with water. You can use juice too, if you like, but don't use carbonated liquids. By putting the glass back in your mouth and leaning your head back, the water will create a liquid simulation of a penis. You will notice that gurgling is relatively difficult once your jaw is locked, and swallowing is nearly impossible. Your tongue will close off your throat. This is another sign that it will only get in the way when you're deep-throating.

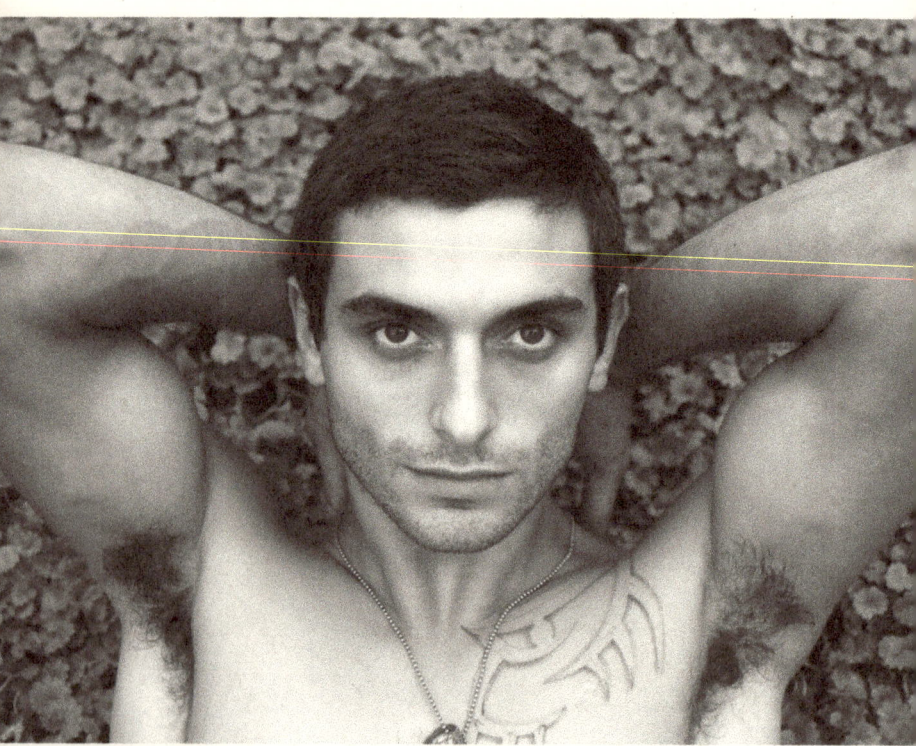

▼ Exercise 3: Banana Blow Job

Now we're getting down to business! Bananas are of course a terrible cliché, but they are actually quite suitable for practicing your blow job skills because they are shaped like an erect penis and have a similar range of variety. Some of them are long and straight, others are small and curved, still others are thick and short, and so on. It doesn't really matter what kind you have to hand, it is sure to have its genital twin somewhere out there. Raw sausages would also be a good option for this exercise, by the way. But personally, the idea of sucking on one really turns my stomach, which is why I would only recommend them if you have a banana allergy.

So let's get started. Before you start giving your banana a blow job, remove the peel. You can leave it on if you like, but who would want to lick a banana peel? The next step should not come as much of a surprise. Just as you did with the popsicle, push the banana back into your mouth as far as possible and hold it there for a moment. This time, you're allowed to gently scrape the surface with your teeth when you pull it out again. This has the advantage of telling you how much of it you have managed to get into your mouth. Logically enough, the rule here is: The further the better. Your other aim should of course be not to break the banana. This also good practice for treating the human banana with care and compassion. From this point on, it's bombs away! Tickle the back of your throat until your eyes fill with tears and try to find out what is too much and what isn't, but also what might actually feel good.

To avoid any misunderstanding: The point of the exercise is not to make you throw up. On the contrary. Your goal is to stop at precisely the point when going any further would make you vomit. When you reach this point the first couple of times, it will be accompanied by the obligatory gagging as well as a shudder running through your entire body, and probably giving you goosebumps or making your nipples hard. After a couple of rounds, you'll notice that you will have started to produce thick, viscous saliva at the back of your throat, which is pulled out in gobbets along with the banana. If this is unpleasant, you can place a couple of paper towels underneath you, but you should also realize that this spit-mucous is highly appreciated by many blow job experts (both tops and bottoms) as an additional benefit. Apart from the fact that it's also a great natural lube. The boundaries between pleasure and disgust can be very flexible. In many cases, moving these boundaries is simply a question of experience.

Moving on. Your banana will not survive much of this treatment for long. Your saliva will soften the surface and it will break off at some point. Before that happens, give yourself a break and eat it. If you feel like going for another round after that, peel another banana and give that one a blow job too. But you should probably stop after three at the most.

Other points to watch out for: Most bananas are curved. When you introduce it into your mouth, try out all four directions—with the tip facing upwards, to the left and right, and facing downwards. The last option is probably the most comfortable for most people, as the downward curve follows the curve of your tongue. But when you're doing the same thing with a real dick, you generally won't be able to choose whether you want it to curve up or down. You can however tilt your face to change the angle and direct the glans into your cheek, for example, instead of down your throat. Practicing the banana blow job in all directions will at least help prepare you for every contingency.

> **Insert it with the tip facing down. The downward curve follows the curve of your tongue.**

▼ Exercise 4: Rubber Bite

Quick test! You will need a freshly washed and dried cucumber for this. Put a condom on it, then follow the standard principle. Stick it in your mouth as far as it will go. In most cases, this will be slightly more difficult than the last exercise, as most cucumbers are thicker than a banana. But what's the rubber for? Simple. First of all, it's to find it whether you can and want to give a blow job with a condom. If you want to be able to use a condom, it's a good idea to test your reactions to the not-always-pleasant taste before you undertake the real thing. Although flavored condoms aren't really my thing, I would strongly recommend using them in this context. The fruity overtones do help cover up the rather off-putting taste of rubber. To be really consistent, go with banana flavored condoms. Secondly, the rubber allows you to safely bite down on the cucumber without breaking the peel. After removing the condom, use your teeth marks to find out your own personal best.

Test results: You know what a blow job with a condom tastes like and you can measure your own personal record in inches. Plus you've familiarized yourself with the cucumber. You'll be using it again for the next exercise.

▼ Exercise 5: Return of the Cucumber

Did I say that practicing blow jobs with vegetables is completely ludicrous? I take it all back. I know, I've already said that, but it took the following exercise to properly convince me. Because this one really is fun. We are going to make our very own blow job penis. Special feature: "fat tip." This will hopefully make the next exercise a bit easier and slightly more realistic. The human dick does not have the same girth as a cucumber. And oral sex is similar to anal in one respect: once you've gotten a prominent glans past the ring of muscle, that's usually half the battle. But first things first: Before we can reach this goal, we've got some chopping and snipping to do. Hold on to the (condomless) cucumber with one hand and, with the other, cut a circle into the peel roughly one inch be-

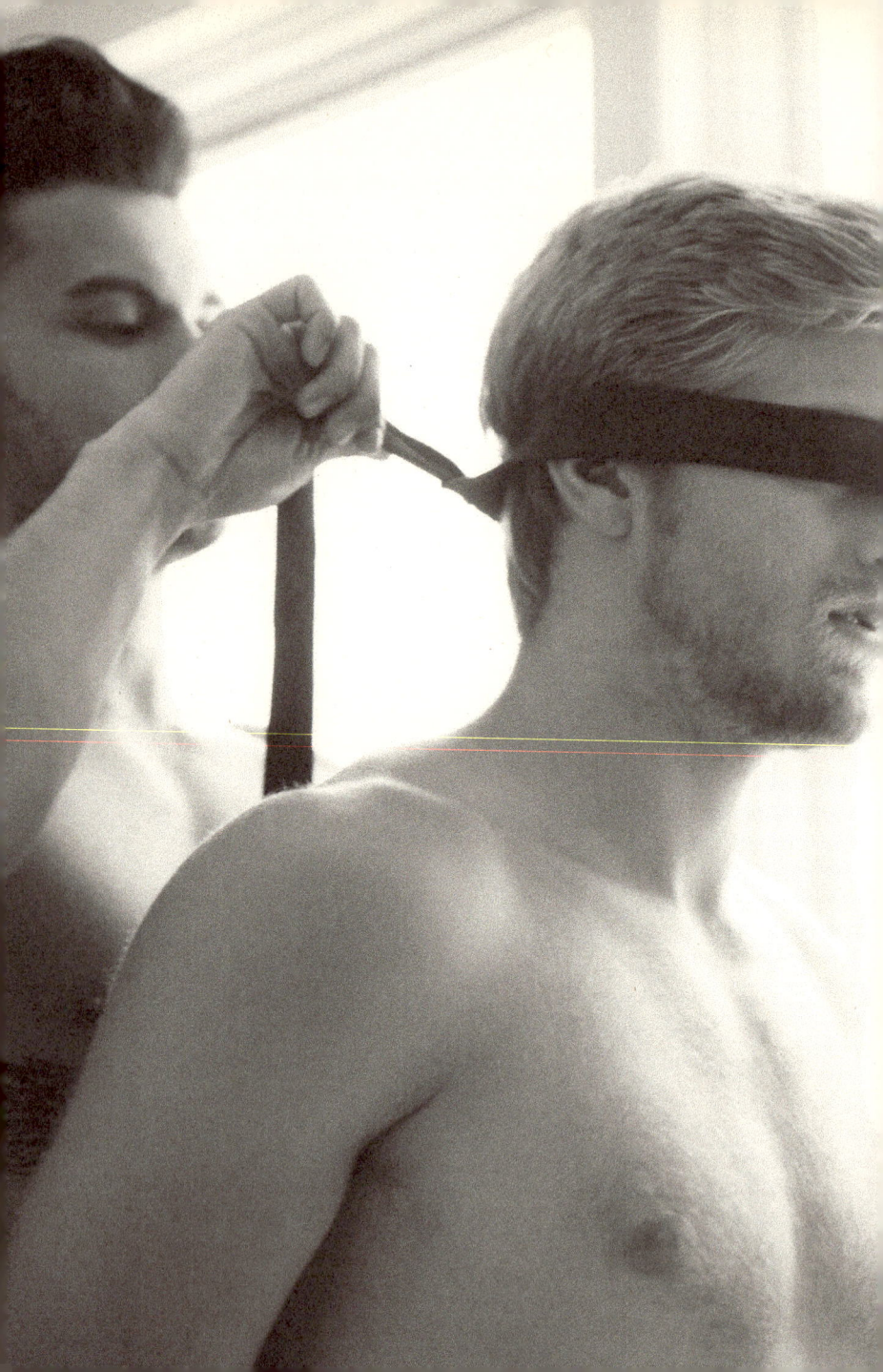

low the tip, using a sharp knife. Don't cut too deep. You don't want the tip to break off. Three millimeters should be enough. Then use the knife to carefully peel the skin off the cucumber, from bottom to top, creating a ridge around the edge of the circle. Or to put it less coyly: One end of your cucumber should look like a wiener with a fat tip. The rest is probably self-evident. Open your mouth, insert the cucumber—with or without a condom—and break your own record. You'll notice that blowing a trimmed down cucumber is much easier than in its natural, uncut state. Try to see this development as a glimpse into the future. Because even though I have finally made my peace with nutritious blow job exercises, I have not changed my mind about them: Once you've given a blow job to a vegetable, you will really appreciate the flexibility of a flesh and blood dick. Which takes us to the last exercise.

> *The DIY vibe is what makes this blow job exercise especially enjoyable.*

Note: If you already possess a realistic dildo, you can sit out the craft session. After all, you've already got a phallus replica, complete with a glans. But let's be honest here: Crafting your own dildo can be a lot of fun and the whole DIY vibe makes the ensuing blow job exercise especially enjoyable. Besides, cucumbers are more slippery and they taste better.

▼ Exercise 6: Now You See Me, Now You Don't

Respect! You've already given a blow job to a popsicle, a champagne glass, bananas, cucumbers, and several condoms. I'm going to assume that you haven't been paying much attention to what your eyes were doing all the while. Were you staring stoically at the ceiling, into the middle distance? Were you watching porn, or were your eyes closed? If it was the latter, you can skip the "Now You Don't" part of this exercise. Because you apparently relied intuitively on your sensitivity and trusted in your blow job instincts.

If this isn't the case, you can use a blindfold to work your way towards this fundamental stance. Keep whatever phallus replica you're most comfortable with to hand and place the blindfold over your eyes. You can close your eyes now, as you won't be able to see anything anyway, and now that you have closed out every conscious and unconscious visual stimulus, you can fully concentrate on holding your breath, finding your gag point and snatching with your lips. Admittedly, blindfolding yourself tends to shift your focus towards your sense of smell, and the lack of any sexually arousing odors among all the bananas, cucumbers and flavored condoms will be sorely noticeable. This should however make you even more aware of how important the smell of pubes and dick sweat is for your sexual pleasure.

When you think you've concentrated enough, you can turn the tables. Now it's time to use the mirror again. Set it up somewhere so that you can watch yourself. Your best option is to lean it against the wall and then get down on all fours and pretend you're giving a blow job to someone lying underneath you. Now watch your facial expressions while you do it. Do you look voracious, or merely strained? Or is your expression aggressive, dedicated, or aroused? To be clear: I'm not asking you to pretend to be turned on in order to look good to yourself! The mirror is not your partner and it is understandably difficult to get excited about blowing fruit and vegetables. But watching your own facial expression will prepare you for sensitive eye contact with your partner later on. Even if it's just a question of remembering to look at him occasionally. You can, of course, replace the mirror with the camera on your phone and watch yourself critically afterwards. Although ... do you really want to film yourself giving a blow job to a cucumber? On the other hand... other people have climbed the dizzy peaks of YouTube fame doing far weirder stuff. So why not?

And now: congratulations! You have successfully graduated from our blow job boot camp. You will know whether it has actually made any difference if you answer yes to at least half of the following questions.

1) Does your room look like a pigsty?
2) Did any part of the training make your eyes water?
3) Did you slobber or slurp at least once?
4) Do you have heartburn?
5) Did you make yourself laugh at least once?
6) Do you feel ready for a real dick (whether out of self-confidence or despair)?

Turn the page for more tips on taming your gag reflex!

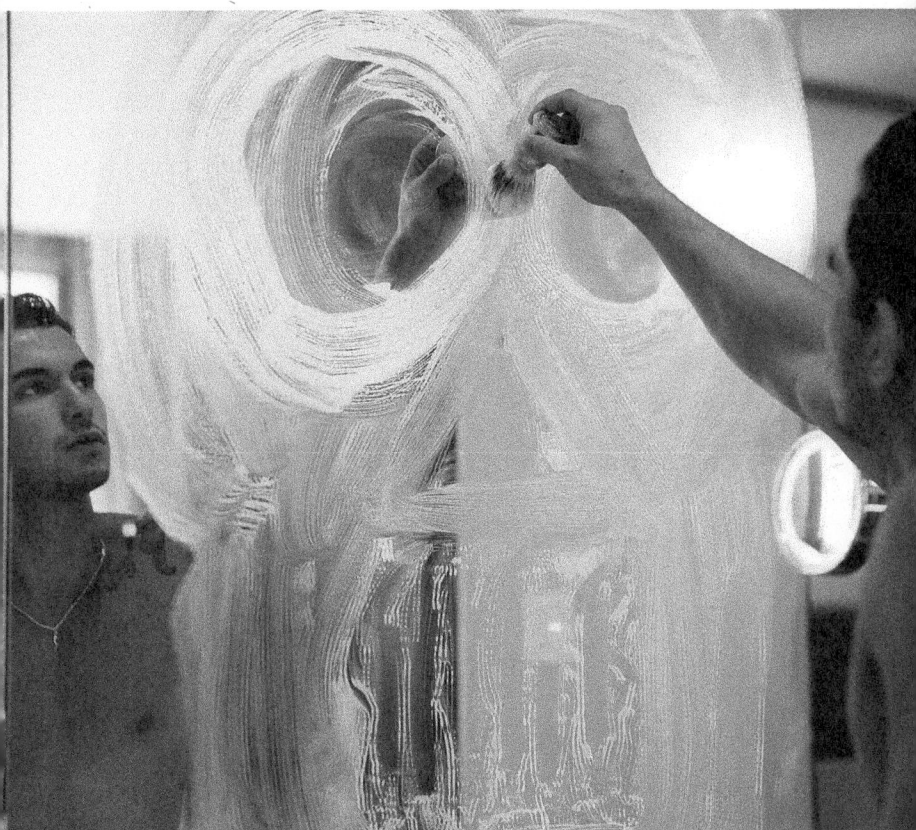

SEVEN TECHNIQUES FOR TAMING YOUR GAG REFLEX

1 – Make a fist
This is more of a placebo distraction maneuver, but it does work to a certain degree. Before you start, fold your left thumb into the palm of your hand and make a fist. Clench and squeeze your thumb for higher deep-throat tolerance.

2 – Numbing sprays or pills
Sprays for numbing your throat are sold in sex shops under names like Blow Job Spray or EZ2SUCK, or available as medication for sore throats from pharmacies as lignocaine or Topex. The active ingredient is generally either lidocaine or benzocaine. The latter is also used in desensitizing gels designed to prevent premature ejaculation. Personally, I'm not a big fan of the scratchy numb sensation that these sprays leave in the back of your throat, so I can't really recommend them, but to my surprise, I have found that they do in fact reduce your gag reflex.

3 – Change position
You can't twist a real dick around like a banana, but you can rotate your own position to accommodate it. At least, as long as your partner is lying down. My point is: If you hit a wall during the classic full frontal blow job, try approaching from the side or upside down (as if you were 69-ing). Sometimes you can thwart your gag reflex simply by adjusting the angle at which the tip of your partner's dick hits your throat.

4 – Swallowing
Swallow before he cums! Or in other words, as soon as you realize your gag reflex is about to kick in, circumvent it by "swallowing" it down. As we saw in our "Seen Through a Glass" exercise, lock-

ing your jaw makes it difficult for you to swallow, but ultimately, this is just a matter of practice. Gina Wild used this technique to become a record-breaking blow job artist.

5 – *The Hummer*
No, this does not involve an SUV—how would that even work? I mean actual humming. The underlying principle is the following: As soon as your partner's glans enters your throat, start humming your favorite tune, and you'll forget all about your gag reflex! Your choice of song doesn't matter so much as the act of humming itself. To avoid sending the wrong signals, you should try to convince your partner that that weird humming sound is actually a purr of contentment.

6 – *Cheating*
If nothing else works, you're going to have to cheat. Making a "cuff" (shortening his penis by wrapping your hand around the root) is one method of avoiding your gag reflex during a deep-throat session. You can also make a tube with your hand (open fist) and hold it in front of your mouth, creating an extension of your oral cavity. Remember to lube your hand up first.

7 – *Hang in there*
You always hated this whenever your teachers said it, but unfortunately, it's true: Practice makes perfect. You've got to realize, the point of the blow job boot camp was to awaken your ambitions and get you to stretch out your antenna. But you will never be a master of the oral arts if you don't repeat the exercises over and over again, and then apply them to your partner on a regular basis!

Get That Dick—How to Do it!

One thing should be clear: Sucking fruit is instructive and fun, but you should always keep your ultimate goal in mind—another man's dick. This is the only way you will ever be able to unlock the secrets of the perfect blow job. Besides, even the most extensive blow job boot camp won't help you if you never try out your newly gained skills on a real man—during a date, while cruising, or with your lover or fuck buddy. The latter are obviously the most intimate and patient test subjects. You can work your way up, inch by inch, and thanks to their constant accessibility, you can also employ the very helpful "blowhard" technique. This means: Take his flaccid or semi-erect wang into your mouth and suck it, moving backwards and forwards and massaging it with your tongue, until it reaches its full size and stiffness. You can generally take in more length this way than if you try and swallow a rock-hard dick. From then on, proceed as you did with the bananas—depending on dick size, keep on deliberately provoking your gag reflex in order to gradually increase your tolerance. Remember to hold your breath as soon as you reach the actual deep-throat point. The frequently recommended technique of breathing through your nose with your mouth full should be used sparingly. It rarely has the effect of allowing to keep going for longer, and instead, frequently results in you having to release your partner's dick sooner than planned. You breathe in

> **The advantages of having a lover or a fuck buddy: intimacy, patience, availability.**

the breaks, whenever your partner's dong slips half-way or fully out of your mouth. Especially as blow jobs rarely consist of keeping a dick in your mouth for minutes on end, as thrusting and letting go constitutes the main attraction. And your breathless panting can be a real turn on for your partner. We'll discuss some of the other go's and no-go's in the next chapter, but now it's time to take a look at some of the various methods for picking up a compatible sex partner. Thanks to online dating and dating apps, it is now extraordinarily easy to find a partner who will not only appreciate your oral skills, but is also explicitly on the lookout for them. But the Internet is only one of four established ways for finding yourself a stud to blow.

▼ Blow Job Dating

Harsh but true: It's not as if the gay world was waiting for you to come along. You'll realize this the moment you enter the search tags "blow job" or "oral" in any dating website. This will get you hundreds of hits, generally from people referring to themselves as "blow job sluts," "bitch faces," "cum whores," and "pussy-mouths"—masses of

> *There's a lot of competition between "blow job sluts" and "pussy-mouths."*

blow job tops looking for bottoms. Or in other words—from the competition. But there's no need to despair. All you need to find a categorical blow job receiver is a little patience and creativity. By using search terms such as "blow me" or "suck me," for example. Or by trawling the quickie profiles according to preference. Or even by ignoring the blow job specific attributes and just going through the profiles of exclusive tops, who generally identify that way because they don't like being penetrated (orally or anally), but who are on the lookout for guys who do. In these cases you will, however, have to have a good think about whether you're prepared to accept an anal addition to your blow job date. Your partner will probably expect this. So if you're not up for that, tell him you're only into blowing him prior to your date. Clear agreements are an important part of fair play. So don't make promises you can't keep and don't bite off more than you can chew. You'll realize that many other people have a very lax approach to this basic principle. This can be pretty frustrating, but it doesn't give you permission to do the same. Always tell

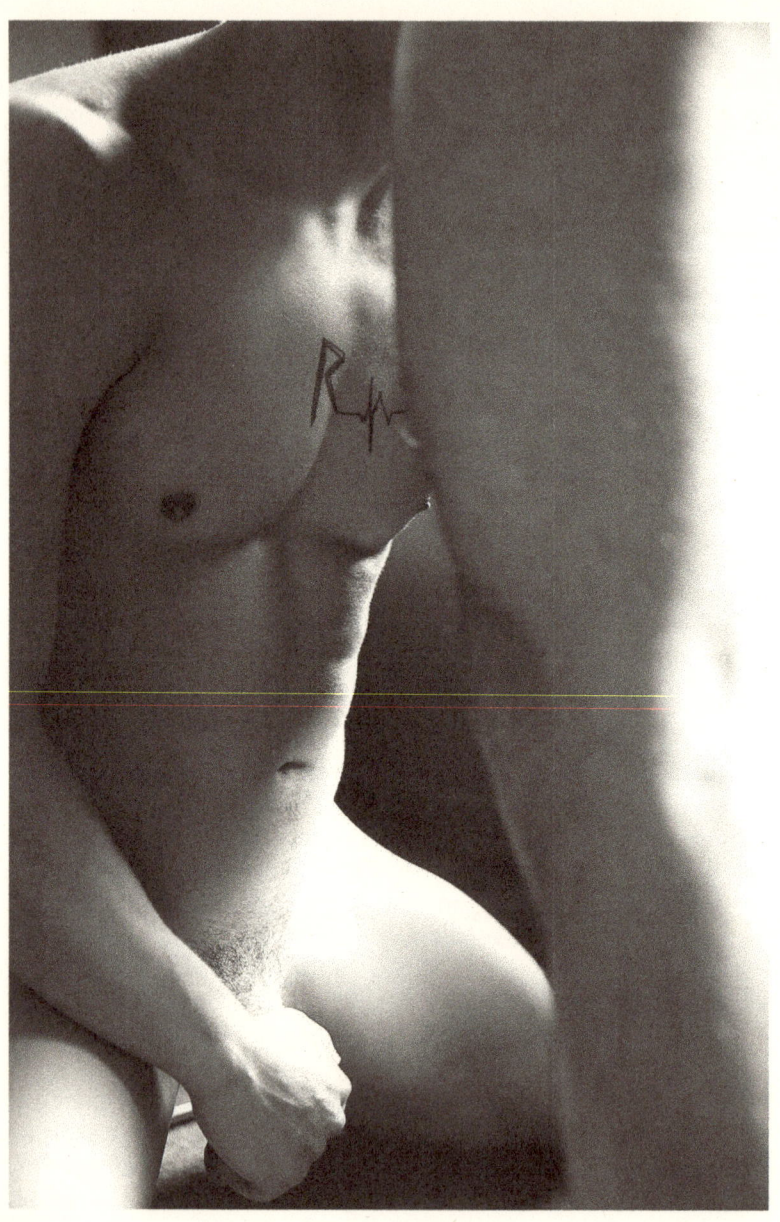

yourself: A guy who lies about his dick size, his preferences, or his safer sex principles in his profile does not deserve a power blow job. The same applies to you. Everything else is a matter of technique, luck, and chemistry. The nicest dick won't do much for you if its owner doesn't know how to use it. But if you like him and he appears willing to learn, you can always take this book along on your second date and suggest he reads the chapter on "Shut Your Eyes!" Getting back to your own online profile: Give yourself an expressive user name, one that allows readers to draw conclusions about your blow job skills and ideally hasn't already been picked by about two thousand other users. This will help interested candidates find you more easily. Upload photos of you that highlight your sexy qualities. Keep those photos up to date. Write a short and concise text expressing what you're looking for. If you're only looking for oral sex and not anal, you should definitely include this in your profile. And when you're chatting, be aware of what you want: You can be friendly, but don't let anyone walk all over you. Anything else can lead to terribly stressful situations.

▼ Blow Job Cruising

If the glory hole marathon described earlier on appeals to you, you'll feel right at home in this category. But you should also realize that you might also be making your life harder than it needs to be. Successful cruising is even more of a question of luck than dating apps. If you hang around saunas, parks or darkrooms waiting for a partner for your next blow job, you will always run the risk of being the only one there. Or of only meeting other blow job tops. Or of turning up after all the nice bottoms have already been taken. In other words: you might need to be more patient and willing to compromise than if you're looking online. Of course, cruising also has its advantages: There's the highly charged atmosphere of a good sex hunt; you have a good chance of being part of a spontaneous group session; and the goods are right out there, in front of your face. Apart from that, the usual mechanisms for making contact are very similar. You will have to conform to the other guy's visual ideals and try and hit the right tone when you chat him up. The general rule is: Most people prefer a spirited approach to indecisive prowling. In addition, you will need to communicate your intentions towards the other guy's dick so that he knows what to expect. Everything else is a matter of willingness and competition. In that order. If your partner gets bored because you're not even trying, there are plenty of other tops lurking on the outskirts who will take him away from you in a flash. To return to the glory hole: Don't believe for a second that all you have to do is position yourself in front of the hole with your lips pursed and wait for one boner after the next to hover into view. Only a few darkrooms feature a clear division, with the tops hanging out on one side and the bottoms approaching from the other. Most glory holes open up into a kind of cabin, which is frequently occupied by people fucking—voyeurs and would-be blow job artists are often seen as a nuisance and blocked off with a T-shirt stuffed into the hole. Use your position as a blow job top wisely and show some initiative instead of sitting down in a corner and waiting for a dick to materialize out of nowhere.

▼ Blow Job Relationships

Long live niche culture! If couples, polyamorous relationships, and fuck buddies are old hat, it's time to introduce a new type of sexual relationship: blow job buddies. This is not entirely serious. After all, it could simply involve two fuck buddies with a preference for oral sex. Relationship models are unlikely to be this explicit. But if they are, I would suggest you reassess your one-trick pony from time to time to avoid misunderstandings. Otherwise, both parties in a relationship that started out as exclusively oral might start to develop a mutual interest in fucking, but because neither of you has ever mentioned it, you will never find out. Even gay men can become creatures of habit, sexually. But you don't have to! The main point of introducing this category is to delineate aspects of the relationship model mentioned above: the friendship with (sexual) benefits. I strongly recommend this model to beginners in particular. There is nothing nicer and more relaxed than exploring your needs and options with someone familiar, someone with whom you can share fantasies without feelings of shame and someone you find attractive enough to want to put these fantasies into practice with him. Apart from the inherent romanticism of this model, it also protects you from emotional hurt or exploitation. This is an enormous advantage in today's cynical and jaded world of gay dating. We are not here to discuss whether stronger bonds may be forged within these kinds of companionable relationships than in a conventional, and still very popular, monogamous relationship, but it is definitely worth thinking about. But if you want to know how to find a blow job partner (or fuck buddy) of your own, all I can tell you is to follow the call of your own instincts. There is no true and tried method. But let me just say this: In a successful relationship, both partners should be equal. Tolerance, trust, security, and a certain degree of sexual attraction are also minimum requirements. You will have to find out for yourself if that is indeed the case. In many cases, all you have to do is overcome your own preconceptions, unrealistic expectations and arrogance. Specifically, the rule "We're buddies; touching is taboo" is not helpful. Nor is the assumption "He's not really my type." Not to mention this attitude: "I'm OK with going out with him, but I only go to bed with really buff guys." Everything else is simply a matter of trying not to compartmentalize. The defining question "We have sex on a regular basis—does that mean we're in a long-term relationship?" should not be in the forefront of your mind. So this involves a lot of hard brainwork—which is easier to do once you've blown away the preconceptions out of your head.

> *Do blow job buddies have more potential than conventional relationships?*

▼ Blow Job Orgies

A bukkake orgy is an organized event combining dating and glory hole strategies. It involves one or several tops sitting in the middle of a circle of bottoms and sucking them off until they squirt jizz onto their faces. You can find any number of clubs devoted to fulfilling this popular sexual fantasy, generally by searching for the terms "gang bang," "sex party" or "bukkake." Apart from a couple of bukkake forums, these very rarely confine themselves to blow jobs. Besides this, these events are not suitable for beginners and you won't even be admitted in most cases if you don't have a certain amount of sexual experience. This is a good thing. If you have only just started out on your blow job career, save this kind of thing for later on when you have gathered enough experience to be able to realistically assess how much you can take, what you want, and how to articulate your needs to others. In other words: Blow job orgies are part of postgraduate studies, rather than an elementary course. They can be a goal, but they are not necessarily part of your journey.

> *Bukkake orgies are more of a postgraduate course than an elementary class.*

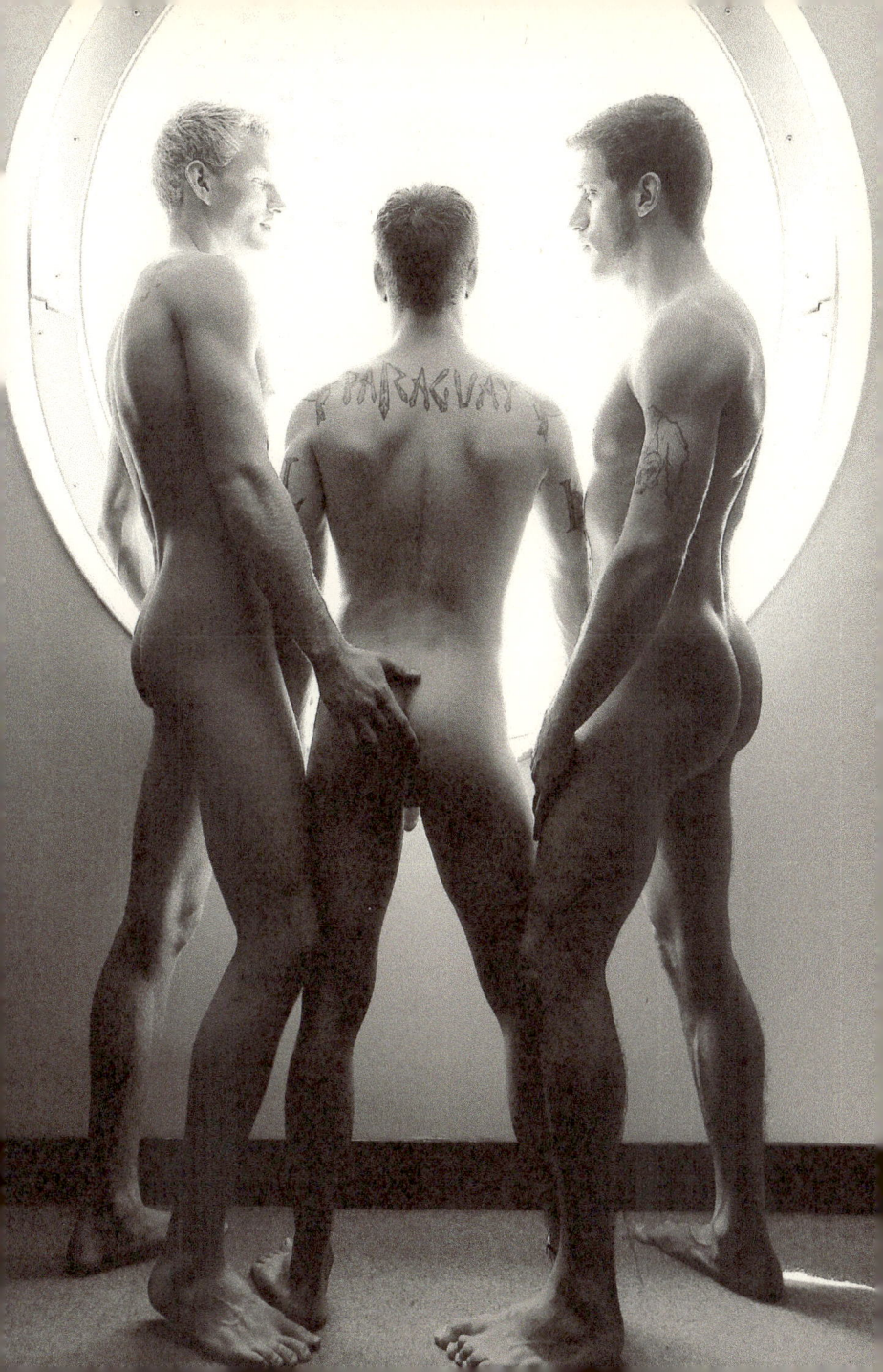

Do's When Giving a Blow Job

1 – Compliments
Guys who like having their dicks sucked tend to be machos at heart. Machos like being complimented—on their smell, their dicks, their hardness ... you'll think of something. Anything goes as long as it's halfway believable. The reverse (even if it's not featured in our list of don'ts) is also true: Never make fun of another guy's body or bodily functions. Even if he has clearly lied about the size of his dick on his profile, be polite. Or if you can't be polite, at least be objective.

2 – Arousal!
Sometimes I get the feeling that blow job artists tend to forget that it takes two to tango. You do have to enjoy giving another man a blow job, but you're not just providing a service! If you want your partner to get hard, it does help if you've got a boner of your own.

3 – Flexibility and Creativity
It's fine if you have your own blow job routine, but you have to be prepared to negotiate. Be open to your partner's suggestions and concentrate on those tricks that he enjoys instead of slavishly following your own routine.

4 – Endurance and Spirit
At the risk of repeating myself: If you get tired after two deep-throats and urge your guy to hurry up and cum, he is definitely not going to enjoy it. Endurance is an important factor. Try and see every blow job as a competition between your own stamina and that of your partner.

5 – Post-Orgasm Service
Whether this point is a must or a no-go is a matter of perspective. What I mean is, if you cum before your partner, don't just stop! Join him on the rest of his journey towards orgasm. If you don't want to go on blowing him, try touching him instead. Unless, of course, he tells you he doesn't want to or need to cum.Es sei denn, er sagt selber, dass er gar nicht kommen will oder muss.

Don'ts When Giving a Blow Job

1 – Bad Eating Habits
This is a two-in-one no-go! In general, stuffing yourself before giving someone a blow job is not advisable. It will simply increase the risk of you throwing up. Besides this, you should always consider your partner before deciding what to eat. If your mouth is still on fire from Sriracha sauce or you've just scarfed up a box of extra strong mints, this can wreak havoc with the sensitive skin of your partner's penis.

2 – Scraping
I cannot stress this enough: Be careful with your teeth. Sure, some people enjoy a gentle nibble around the shaft or the foreskin, but nobody likes thrusting back and forth with their partner's teeth scraping down the length of their cock. Besides which, this can easily cause injury.

3 – Surprises and Force
Surprises: Unless you're enjoying a quickie and pressed for time, sudden deep-throating can be a bit too much for your bottom. Take your time. Forcing yourself: If you would rather not do something, then don't do it. Politeness does not involve sucking an unappetizing dick.

4 – Distraction and Self-Centeredness
As I already mentioned on the Do's page, you are not a service provider. This is true. But neither is your partner. Even if using and being used is consensual, you still need a certain amount of dedication. If you can't concentrate on what you're doing, do something else.

5 – Post-Orgasmic Insatiability
Pushy blow job devotees who go on snatching at their partner's dong—even while he's heaving in the throes of orgasm—are the worst. Sure, some BDSM practices do involve playing with your partner's sensitivity. But for most people, this grabby kind of behavior is a real turn-off.

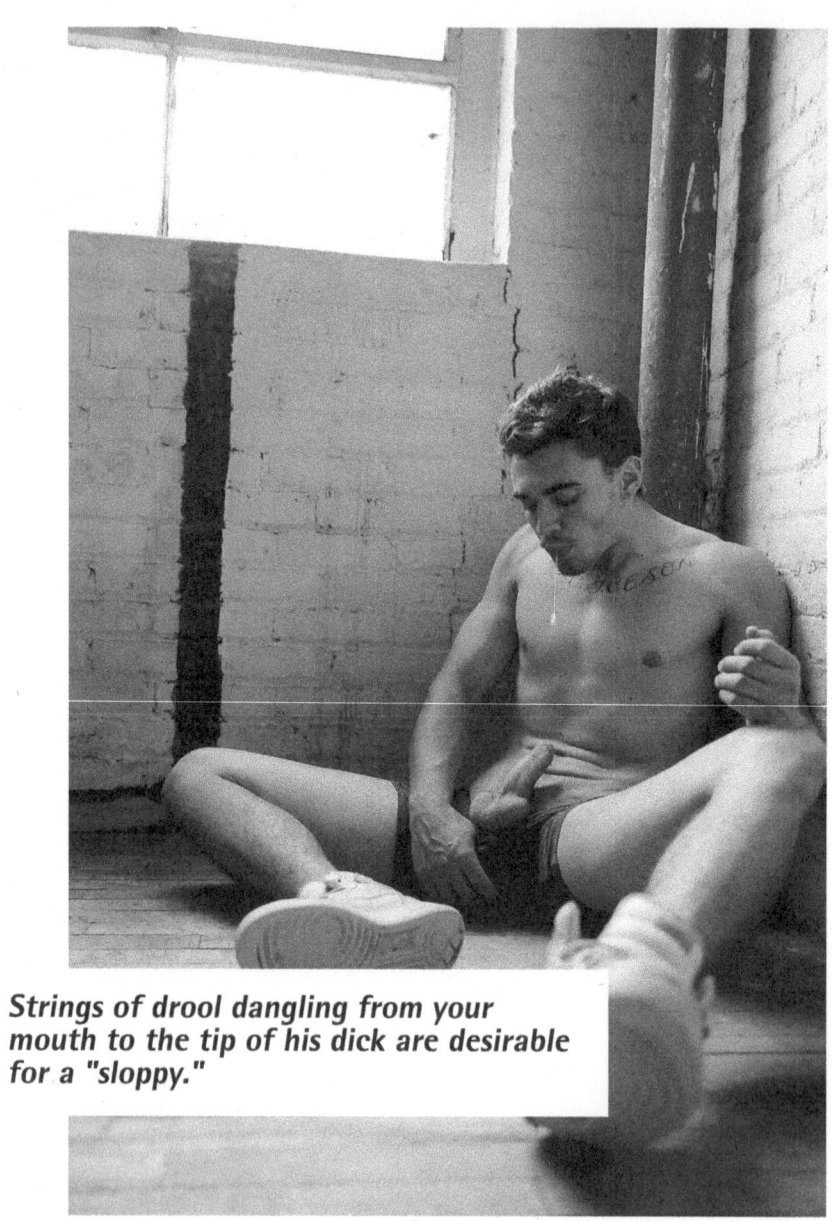

Strings of drool dangling from your mouth to the tip of his dick are desirable for a "sloppy."

The Triumph of Technique—Blow Job Methods for Tops

▼ Sloppy Style

One man's "yuck" is another's mouthwatering deliciousness. The sloppy blow job is one of the more Rabelaisian techniques—cast off your inhibitions and slurp, squelch, and drool to your heart's content. This is, to a certain extent, the epitome of good oral sex job, as the best blow job is always wet. If you deny that, I doubt you've ever really had one. As even casting off your inhibitions takes practice, choose a suitable environment for your first sloppies, one where you won't have to worry about making a mess—whether it's outdoors, inside a sex club, or even your own (tiled) bathroom. Of course, you can also follow the example of many watersports enthusiasts and just put down a waterproof liner on your living room floor. This does however interfere with spontaneity. On the other hand ... does it matter? Most of us have been aware that dribbling and slobbering are generally considered inappropriate for at least two decades, so ditching this rule doesn't necessarily have to be spontaneous. To get back to the action: As I said, the point of this exercise is to get your juices flowing. Strings of drool dangling from your mouth to the tip of his dick form part of the attraction of this variation, and occasional spitting is inevitable. It goes without saying that this generally goes hand in hand with passionate deep-throating.

▼ The Gimmick Blow Job

Speaking of sloppy: Does anyone remember the grapefruit blow job demonstrated by American fellatio expert Auntie Angel, whose YouTube clicks reached dizzying heights in the spring of 2014? What makes this technique so spectacular, according to the sex educator, is the fact that it gives the bottom the illusion of fucking and being sucked off at the same time. Millions of Internet users were intrigued, and so the video starring Auntie Angel trimming off both sides of the grapefruit, cutting a dick-sized hole into the pulp, placing it over a dildo and performing oral sex on it, went viral from day one. If you've ever tried it out yourself, you'll probably agree that it's not really that close to fucking-and-being-sucked-off-at-the-same-time and that the whole thing is unbelievably sticky and messy. But it's a very creative idea all the same. It's also a classic example for the gimmick blow job. Instead of a grapefruit, you can also use rice, piercings, ice cubes, vibrators, or cock rings to spice up your blow job. I'll go into these in more detail in the chapter on "Bonus Material" on page 104. At this point, I'll confine myself to advising you not to jump the gun when it comes to hauling out the gimmicks. It's better to explore your own and your partner's individual blow job needs and preferences before you start getting fancy. Once you're familiar with your partner's preferences, you can choose and employ any gimmicks according to their needs.

▼ Lip Service

This kind of blow job can be easily boiled down to a single instruction: Leave your tongue out of it! Instead, concentrate on providing wraparound service with your lips. If your partner has a foreskin, pull if forwards and use both lips to massage the glans through the foreskin with a side to side motion. (If he doesn't have a foreskin, this move is only advisable if your lips are exceedingly soft and well-lubricated.) Employ the snatching movements mentioned in our boot camp to work your way up his boner with your lips and add targeted pressure in places to massage the tissue. In brief: Leave everything you would otherwise do with your

Giving head without using your tongue is the oral version of "look, no hands!"

tongue (licking across the shaft, tickling the glans, creating tiny vibrations etc.) to your lips. You will soon see how inventive you can be if you're forced to concentrate on just one element. The

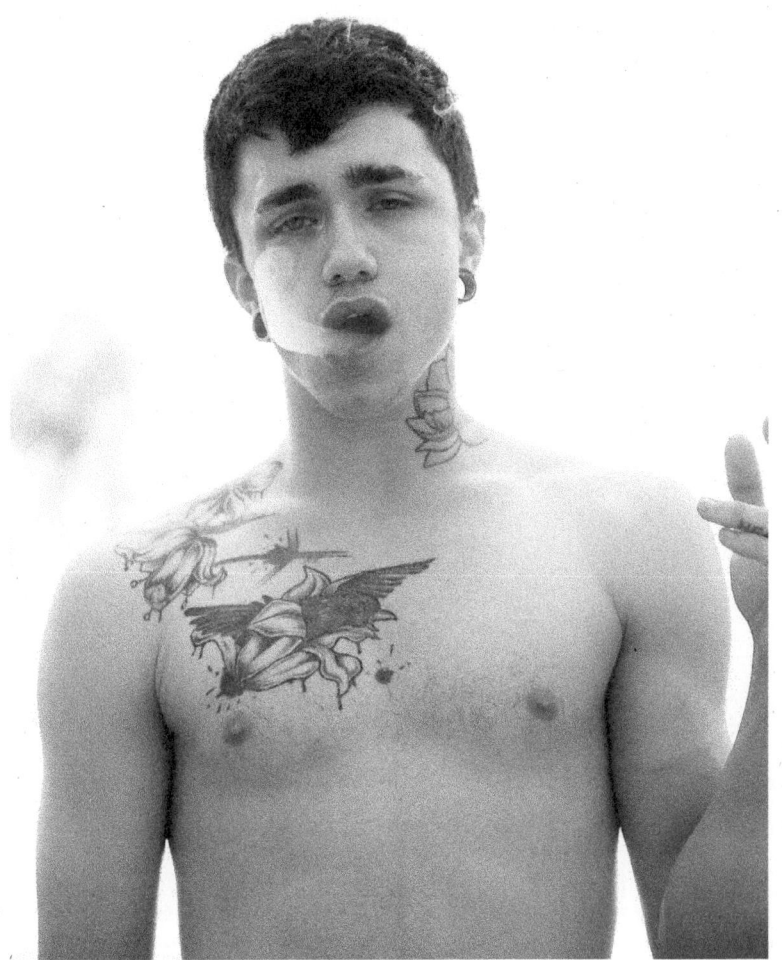

same principle can also be applied to the "Look, No Hands!" exercise. The latter does however put quite a strain on your sense of balance, agility and patience, and can quickly turn into a chore for the bottom.

▼ The Submissive

It takes a lot of self-assurance and confidence in your own skills to utter the words "Use me!" You can't let yourself be used if you don't know how you work. You also need a trustworthy partner who can be relied on to handle this request responsibly. You need to have reached quite an advanced level to give someone a really submissive blow job. But if you're ready for this level, it can be extremely hot. It entails passing control over to your partner and letting him determine the action. An experienced partner will know how to use this privilege, while at the same time always remembering to ask himself whether you need a break. This is essential, as there is no point in letting yourself be used if you're not enjoying it. You can, of course, help fan the flames by begging for his dick.

▼ Blind Man's Buff

In one of our boot camp exercises, we used a blindfold to screen out visual stimuli and enable us to concentrate fully on the sensations of giving a blow job. The same principle makes even more sense when you reverse it. You can carry on using your blindfold outside of the boot camp exercises by blindfolding your lover—ideally as soon as the action between his dick and your mouth starts to pick up speed. To avoid losing his balance, your partner should be seated on the edge of the bed and support himself with his hands behind him. Kneel down between his legs, spit on his boner, and massage it slowly with your hands. Flick your tongue over the glans, go on massaging him, take the tip between your lips, release it, and continue massaging him while gradually increasing the intensity. Using the breaks to announce what you're about to do next can also be very effective. This will create expectations, increasing the suspense and pleasure for both of you. I do realize this is starting to sound a bit *Fifty Shades of Grey*, but if you're both so turned on that you talk like that without feeling stupid, you can create an unforgettable experience for your partner.

▼ Torture

There are many ways of pleasurably torturing your partner during sex, and few very sex acts are as well suited to this procedure as the blow job. Unlike during anal sex, for example, you can completely take over during oral sex. For example, by having your partner lie on his back, you can lean over him and work on his junk without him being able to do much about it. But you can also

> *His dick will go off like a fountain after you've tortured him for a while.*

"torture" him just as well while he's standing or sitting down. As you may have suspected, this isn't about causing him actual pain, but instead making him a slave to his own pleasure. Turn him on and then... make him wait. Bend forwards and suck his glans, then take it into your mouth briefly, but only until he starts purring with pleasure, and then, the moment he stops expecting it, you pounce and give him the mother of all blow jobs until you can feel he's about to cum. Then stop again and torture him by depriving him of his orgasm. If you stick to your guns and don't let up, his dick will go off like a fountain the moment you let him cum.

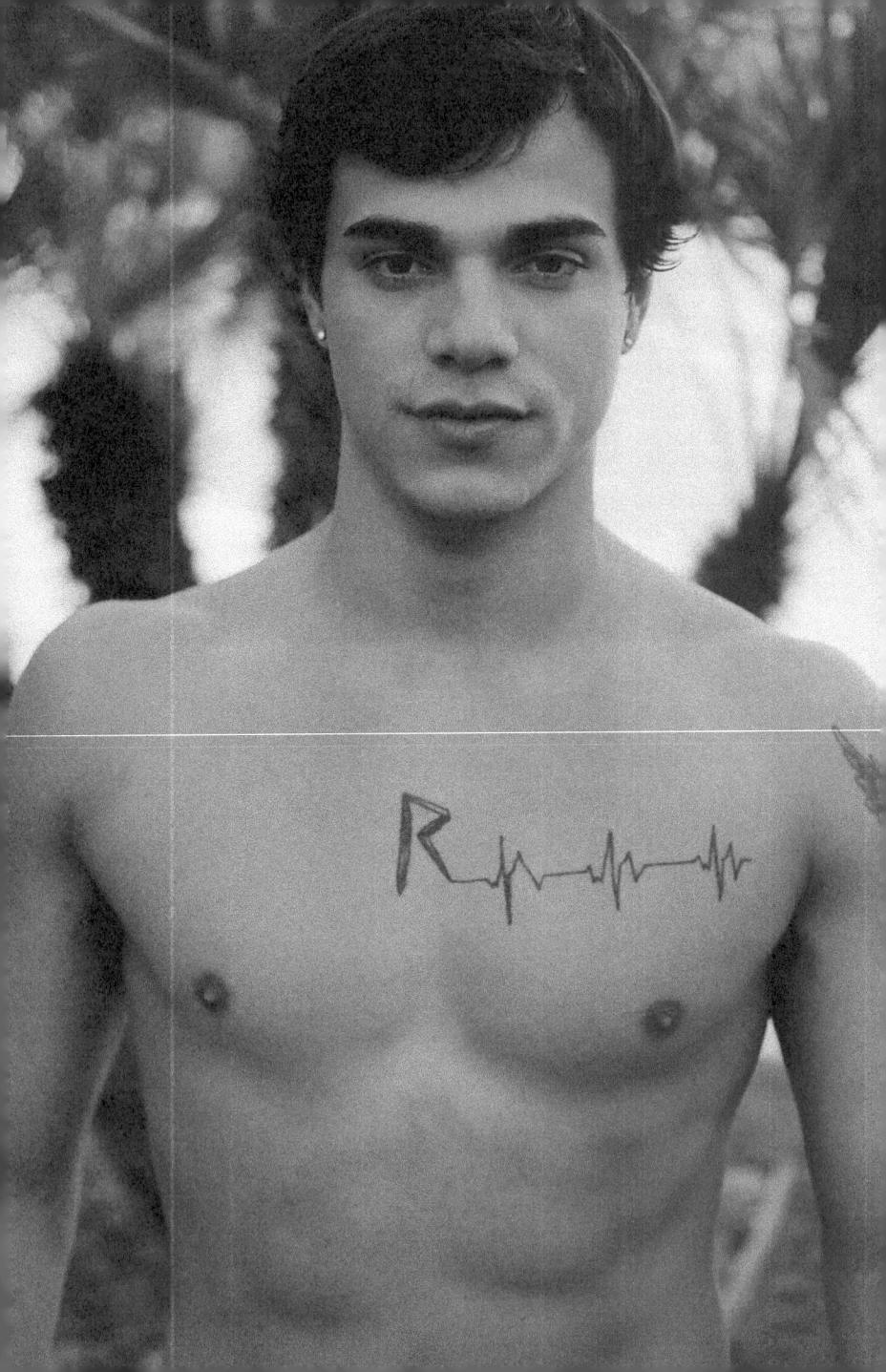

Interview with CockyBoys Blow Job Top Levi Karter: "No Love, No Blow Job"

At the comparatively tender age of twenty-three, porn idol Levi Karter has already had an eventful life. He has both topped and bottomed, acted and directed, and starred in solo scenes and double penetration sessions for his regular label CockyBoys. He is a natural born porn star. But his one true passion is oral sex. Which is why we've called him in for an expert's opinion!

When was your first blow job, and what was it like?
That was with my very first boyfriend. I had just turned fifteen and I was a top, of course. I loved it from the word go.

When did you realize you preferred giving blow jobs to receiving them?
I'm not sure when exactly, but it was pretty early on. I think it's because knowing I'm making my partner feel good really turns me on. I'm generally more of a giver than a taker.

What qualities do you need to give a blow job?
Practice and especially affection. I think you need to feel a certain amount of love for a really dedicated blow job.

Any expert tips for aspiring blow job artists?
I'd say, the most important this is to keep your breathing under control. Sometimes this entails holding your breath. If you're deep-throating, for example, you shouldn't breathe at all, not even through your nose. If you don't have a partner, you can practice with a dildo. The same applies if you do have one, but giving head makes you drool and gag. Unless your partner is into that. If you're using a dildo, make sure it's not ridiculously oversized.

What is your opinion on the following theory: "Oral sex is not just foreplay, it's a whole category of sex in itself"?

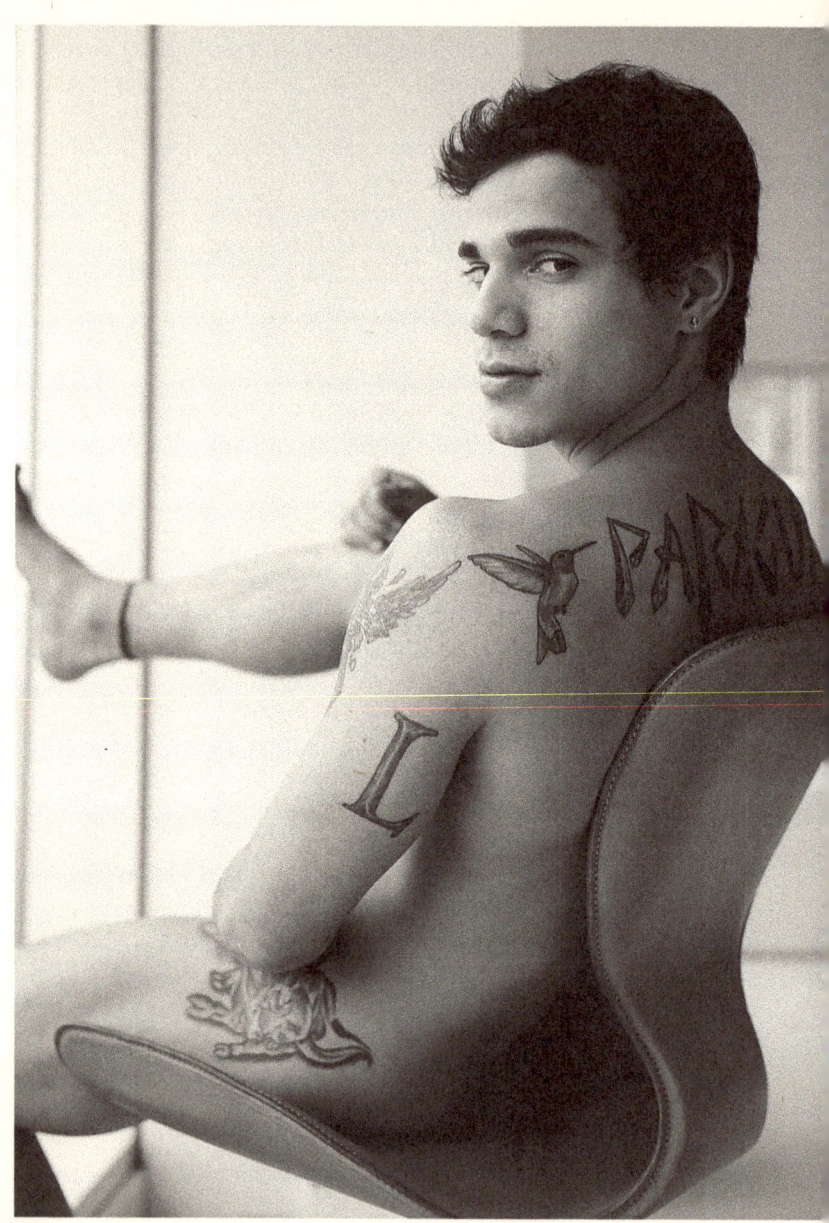

I agree wholeheartedly. In my opinion, oral sex allows you to enjoy each other just as much as anal. Maybe even more. It depends on the situation. For me, it also depends on the kind of chemistry I have with my partner.

How do you tell which blow job techniques work best with a guy and which do not?

Try everything out and observe closely. If in doubt, I use all the techniques I know and offer the bottom a buffet of possibilities. You generally know what works and what doesn't before you've completed the first round. Some guys like you swallowing them up to the hilt and keeping them there, others are happy with you sucking the glans and stroking the shaft at the same time. Their reactions to one technique or another will quickly tell you what direction to move in.

What part of oral sex do you enjoy the most?

I like swallowing a really hot, semi-erect dick up to the hilt and feeling it throbbing and growing inside my mouth.

And the other way round? What constitutes a real turn-off?

Well, they do need to be clean. After all, I put them in my mouth. *[Laughs]*

The greatest challenge during oral sex?

I would say concentrating. It's always shitty when my mind starts wandering, but that's partly because I have ADHD. Communicating your needs always presents a new challenge. It never feels good if you have trouble getting your partner to understand what you want.

What kind of thing do you appreciate most in a bottom?

Personally, I like them to be dominant. A guy grabbing my head and pressing it down firmly on his cock—that turns me on.

Is there such a thing as a dick that's "too big"?

For me? No! *[Laughs]*

Is there any difference in how you handle a small dick and a large one?
That happens automatically. Some dicks just aren't big enough for deep-throating. They only reach as far as your throat. Others, on the other hand, can be too thick to take into your mouth at first. You have to use your intuition to adapt to the situation.

Your most notable blow job accident?
No idea. I recently got an eyeful of semen. Does that count as an accident? *[Laughs]*

What are your views on the fetishization of "facials" [cumming in someone's face] and swallowing semen?
I love both of them. But I generally don't swallow if I've already cum myself.

True or false: "There are too many cocksuckers in the world of gay men"?
False. You can never have too many cocksuckers.

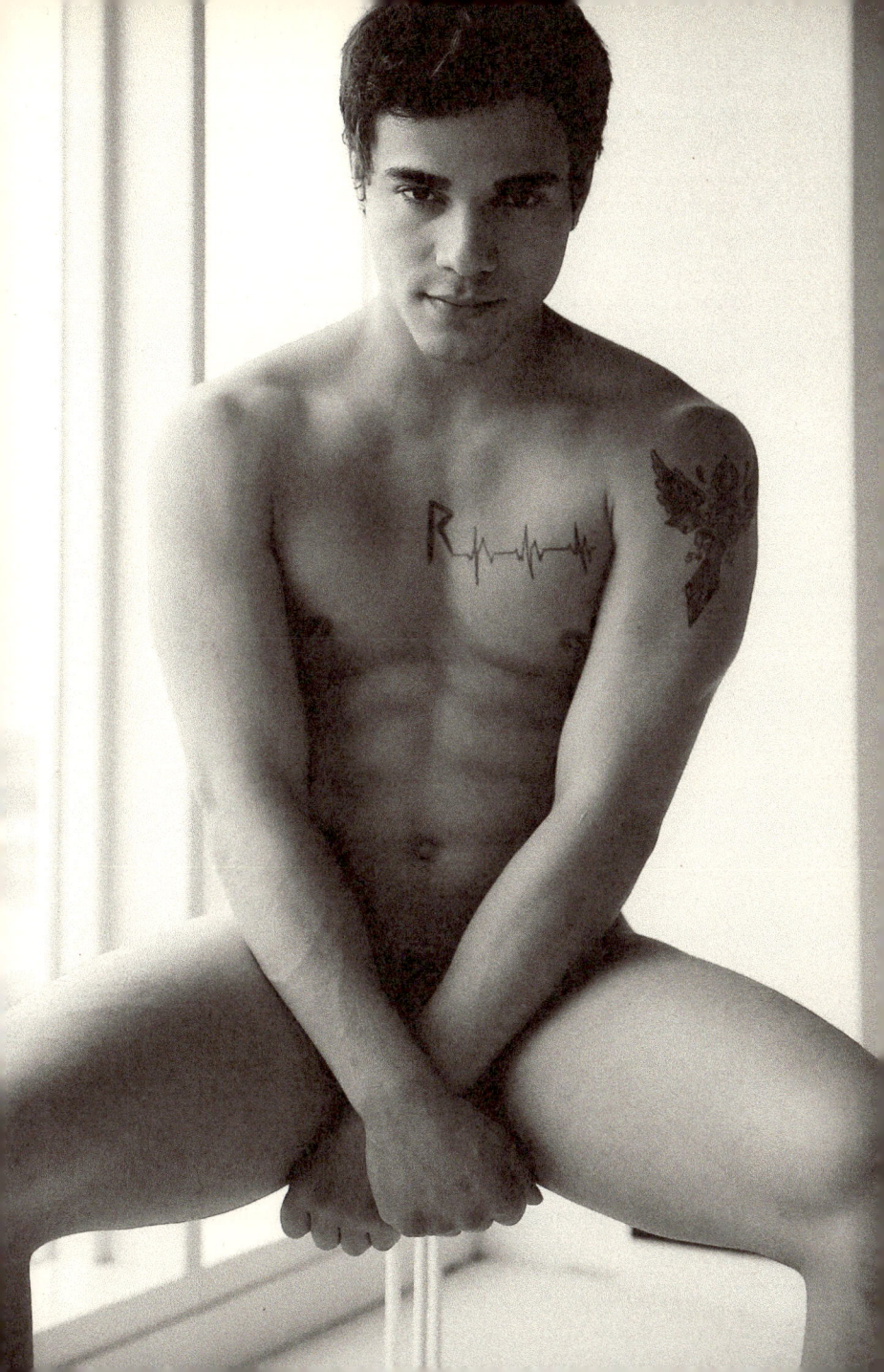

Bonus Material: Blow Job Toys for Tops

▼ Mouth Guard

No, you don't have to go and see your dentist for a custom-fitted mouth guard. You can also get the kind used by boxers from a sports goods store. These are available in a variety of shapes and sizes. Some of them are thick and unwieldy, but the slimmer models will not only help you keep your teeth in check if you have trouble with this during oral sex. They can also produce interesting sensations for the bottom.

▼ Piercings

Piercings, whether through your lips or your tongue, can be integrated nicely into a blow job for a little extra tingle. Vibrating "tongue bullets," with a structured surface, were designed for that very purpose. Hot. But always make sure there are no sharp edges.

▼ Cock Rings

Not every bottom is constantly prepared, not to mention professionally equipped, for a rendezvous with your mouth. So why not keep a couple of cock rings in different sizes on hand to surprise your partner with. And for your own enjoyment, of course. Cock rings (placed over the root of the bottom's penis to block the blood flowing out of his erect dick) will make his cock thicker and make the veins stick out. This feels great for tops. But always remove the ring after an hour at the most.

▼ Blowing Hot and Cold

Sucking an ice cube before or during oral sex will turn your oral cavity into a deep-freeze and create a special challenge for your bottom. Whether or not he enjoys it will depend on your partner.

Not everyone is into "blow jobs on ice" and even the strongest erection may wilt under this treatment (the cold makes the blood vessels dilated during an erection contract), but if he's sufficiently turned on, the feeling of slight numbness that ensues in the aftermath can be very exciting. You can extend this by applying hot and cold treatments, which entail spitting out the ice cube and warming up your mouth with some hot tea. Not too hot—you don't want to burn yourself. Sucking on an ice cube will also leave your mouth slightly numb.

▼ Rice, Tic Tacs & Co.

Experiment with textures! Stuff a handful of Tic Tac mints, mini gummi bears or a spoonful of (boiled) rice into your mouth before performing oral sex on your partner for an unfamiliar tingling sensation. Careful: This method is more complicated for tops than it sounds. You will have to stick to gentle sucking and flicking with your tongue. High speed blow jobs are a choking risk.

▼ Food for Thought

Jelly, Nutella, ketchup, and cream—anything that can be spread or smeared around can also be applied to a boner and licked off again. If you want to turn your lover into a lollipop, and he's into it too... go crazy! Be careful with anything really sticky, though. In addition: As we already mention in our list of Do's and Don'ts, some guys are too sensitive to enjoy hot sauce or breath mints applied to their junk. For others, however, it's quite the reverse. Many couples swear by Altoids and Sriracha. But please proceed carefully.

▼ Spreader Gags

A tool for hardcore kinksters. If you want to restrain your own snapping muzzle or have a partner who prefers to play it safe, you can use a spreader gag or ring gag. Both of them incorporate a steel

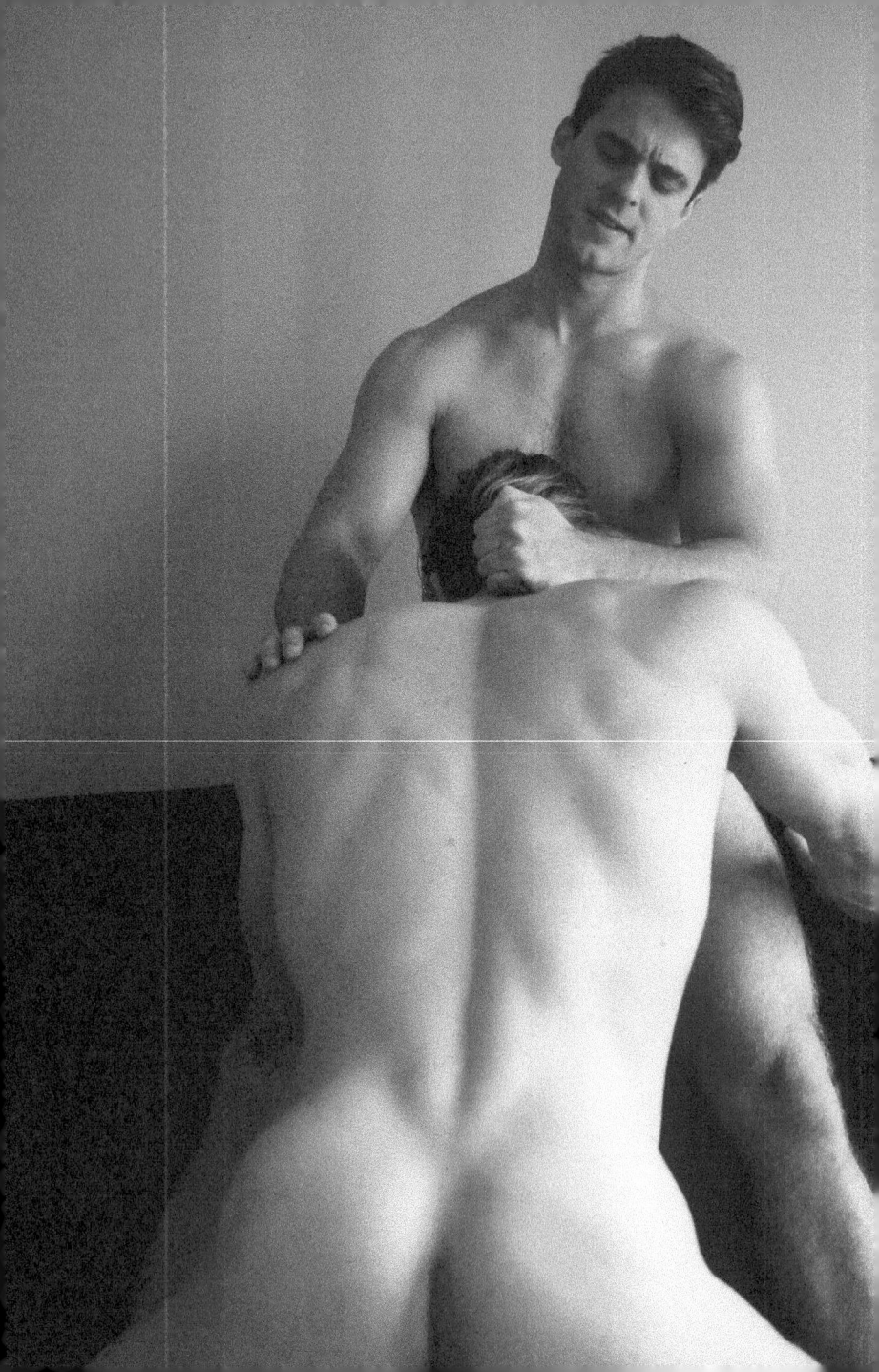

ring or frame that prevents the wearer from closing his mouth. These are also sometimes used during dental surgery and many of them also feature a tongue depressor, which pushes the tongue down into the lower jaw. This frees up even more space for the bottom. Spreaders should only be used with a trusted partner. And you have to want that feeling of help-lessness, otherwise it's horrible. One more thing: As the spreader also prevents you from swallowing, it will make you drool buckets. You should be prepared for this as well.

> *The spreader prevents you from swallowing. You will drool buckets.*

▼ Dildos

An optional toy, useful for everything and nothing. You can pass the dildo to your partner and tell him to use it on you while you suck him off, or you can use it yourself, either as an alternative to your partner's dick, or to conquer his ass ... everything is possible, nothing is mandatory.

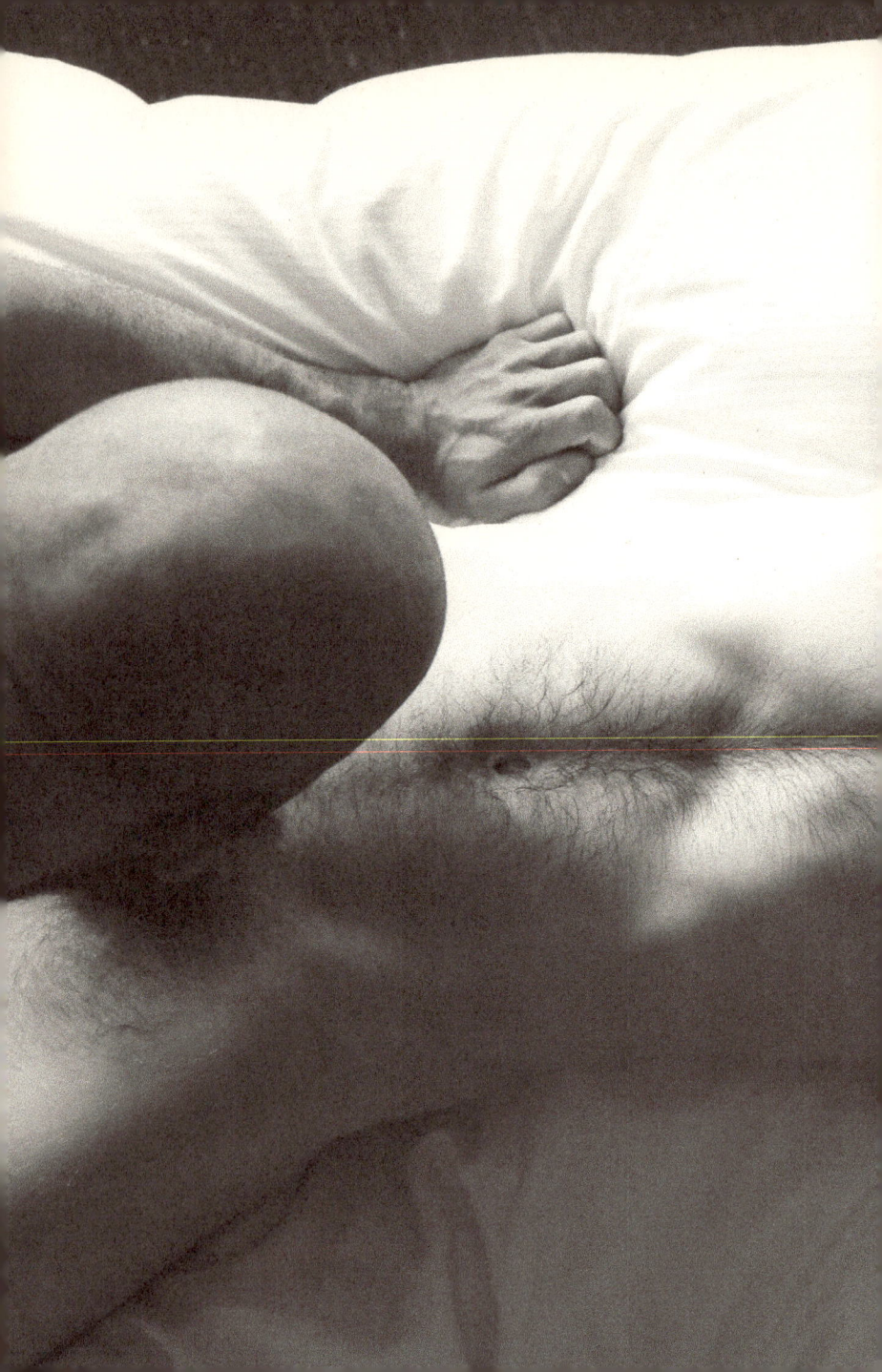

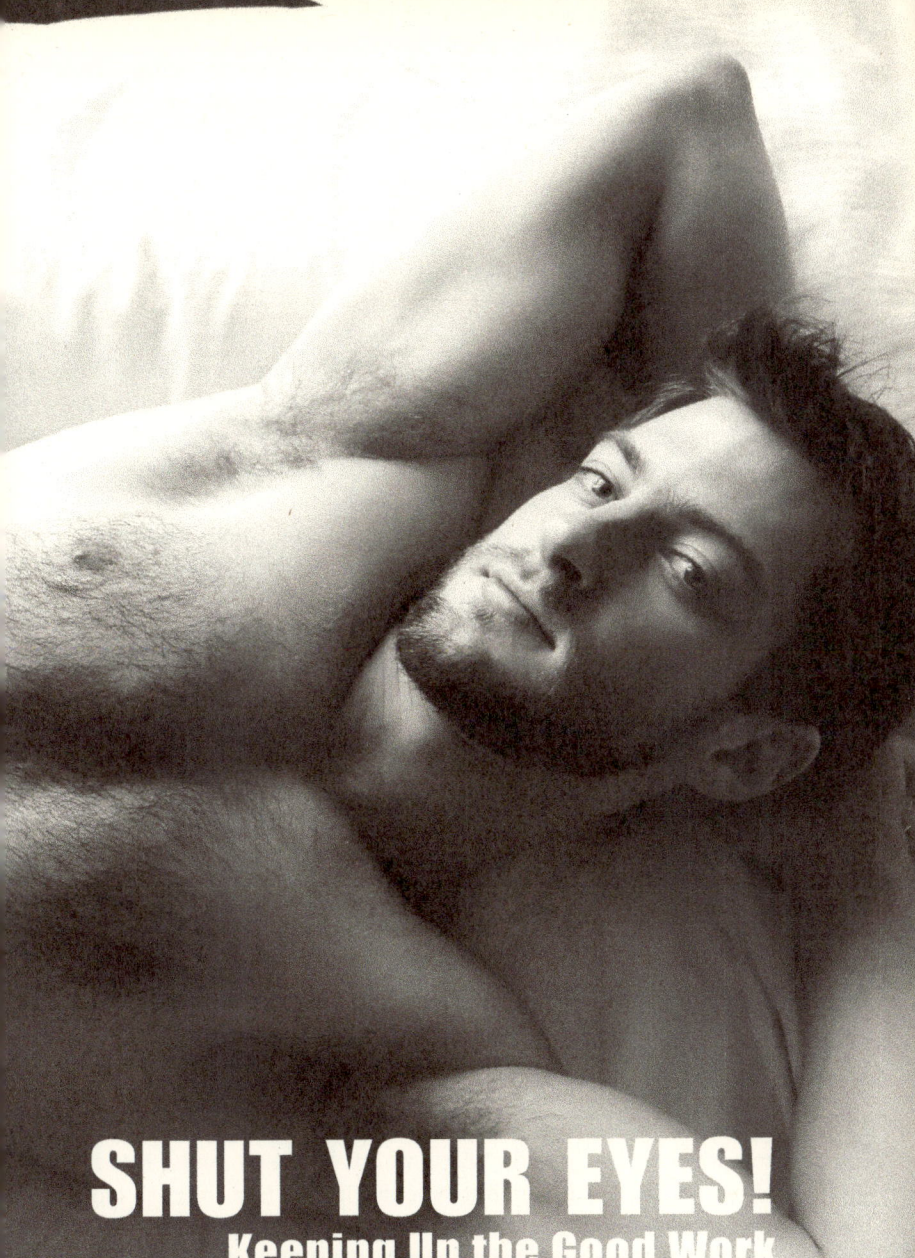

Shut Your Eyes!

Basic Positions: Standing to Attention

Your dick's on fire and the only way of putting it out is by plunging it into your sex partner's mouth as often as possible. That's great! The world of gay men loves a guy like you. Sweeping statements such as this are fine to begin with. But let's take a more nuanced look. Of course, it's not enough to just be constantly hot for a mouth fuck; you also need to know how to control and use that hotness. It takes technical know-how to control it and respect for your sex partners to use it properly. We will be working on both of these things in the following chapters. When I say "Shut Your Eyes!", that doesn't mean you should just lean back and tune out. We are going to take a good self-reflective look at the mechanisms behind receiving a blow job, but we are also going to apply some practical training. And the best way to take a look at something and to practice it is to keep your eyes open. And your mind as well. So we're going to start off by standing up!

The nice thing about receiving a blow job is that you are never in the wrong position. While the top has to bend, squat or kneel down, we can just stay where we are—lying down, sitting, or standing up—and let him do his thing. As long as the earth doesn't literally move, there isn't much for you to do. And if we do occasionally feel like showing a bit more initiative, we can just flip him onto his back and pound him from above. Living the dream! But of course it can't hurt to take a look at the advantages of a range of positions, and pick our own personal favorite. A first self-reflective step in the right direction!

> *While the top has to bend, squat, or kneel down, the bottom is always in the right position.*

Standing up: This is really the best position for receiving a blow job. You can gaze down at your top, stand with your legs slightly apart for more stability, and you've even got your hands free in case you want to stroke your partner's head or give it a push. Or for a real macho stance, you can even drink an ice-cold beer or smoke a cigarette. Stand your ground.

On your back: For epicures and lazy people. There are two options here: You can lie flat on your back with your arms outstretched and just let your partner pamper you, or you can prop yourself up on your arms behind you with your legs dangling over the edge of the bed. As I'm trying to get you to put in some effort at least, I would like to suggest the second option. Our sex partners deserve our undivided attention while they're providing for our needs. This is easier to do when you're propped up. Besides the fact that your mind tends to stray if you're lying flat on your back like a turtle.

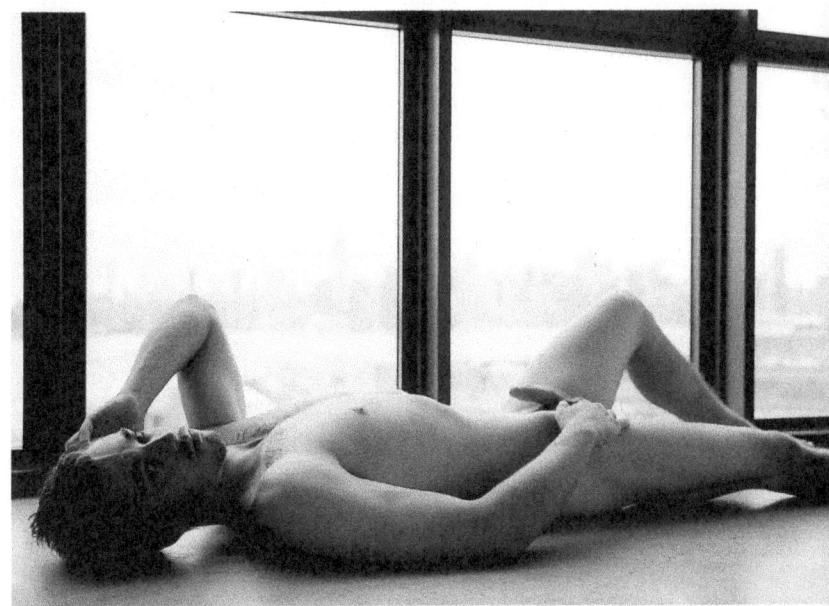

Sitting down: While this position is only ideal if you sit down on the edge of a chair or the bed with your legs spread, sitting bolt upright rarely gets you in the mood. Sitting down is really more of a top position. There's a reason why blow jobs given from under the desk usually end in a standing ovation.

The push-up: Sounds like hard work! And that's what it is. If you do assume the push-up pose with your partner lying on his back underneath you in and your junk in his mouth, you're either going to need strong arms or you'll have to turn onto your side very soon. In other words: a crossover position. In my experience, the only time you ever switch over to this position is when you start out lying down. But blow jobs rarely end that way. After all, an orgasm is hard work in itself.

On your side: Perfect for 69-ing, but not for anything else. Unless you bend one of your legs and use your hips to add momentum, this position is a bit like being asleep with your eyes open. Neither one thing nor another. But it is pretty comfortable.

Ultimately, only one thing counts: It has to be relaxed and enjoyable. Apart from that, a lot of this depends on the situation. You won't have the same energy levels to expend on a blow job on a Sunday morning after a long Saturday night as you will on a frisky Friday evening. And even that depends on your surroundings. The main point of the ideas delineated above is to make you more aware of how your position while receiving a blow job can affect your enjoyment. So if you realize you're simply not getting into it or can't concentrate, try changing positions! Or try them all out right now for a quick jerk-off session to explore their respective advantages and disadvantages. Once you've done that, you've earned yourself a short break, which you can use to go shopping with the following list (you will need all the utensils on the list for our upcoming blow job boot camp), or you can move on to the next theoretical lesson and identify your dick type. Turn the page!

BETTER SHOPPING: A SHOPPING LIST FOR BOTTOMS

- melon

- feathers

- lube

- fake fangs

- a handheld mirror

- condoms

- knife

- paper towels

- glasses

If you haven't got one, now is the time to invest in a (not too large) fake mouth. You can always use an extra mouth.

- masturbator

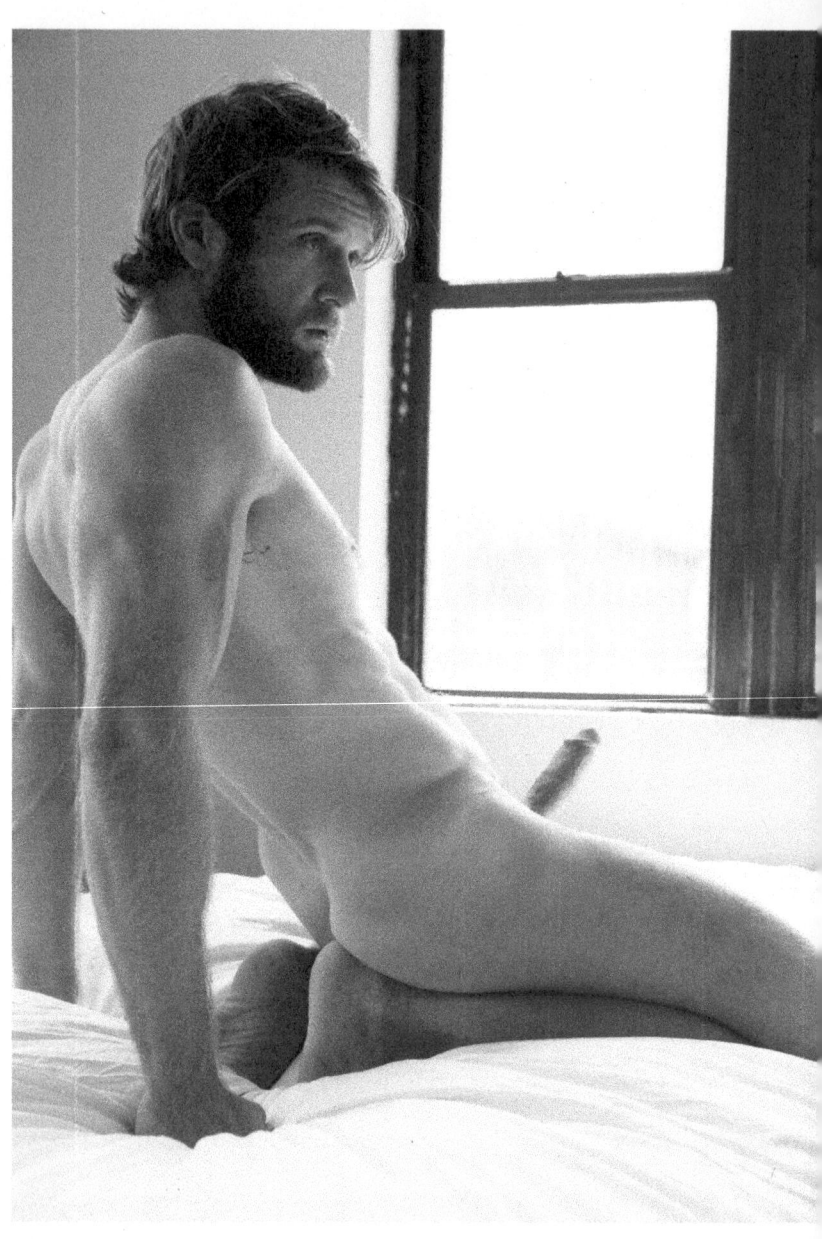

What's Your Dick Type?

No two dicks are the same and no two blow jobs are the same. Nevertheless, as soon as you start engaging with your own sexuality, you will develop certain preferences and specialties over time, all of which will have an influence on your relationship with your cock. This may also include letting go of certain fantasies because they simply don't conform to your own temperament or anatomy. Letting go of an impossible fantasy may be disillusioning, but it should also mark the beginning of a more honest and intimate relationship with your genitals. So let's be honest, gentlemen, and take a look at what part our dicks play in the formation of our personalities—ideally, it should be a little of everything.

▼ Humpers

Satisfying your urges is more important to you than taking good care of your dick. The latter is robustly built and can take a lot of punishment, but also demands a lot of attention. In other words: It keeps trying to take over your everyday life by surprising you with constant, random erections, which has proven quite a successful tactic. If you are still young and in the first bloom of manhood, this is totally normal. If you've just come out and are currently exploring the benefits of man-on-man sexuality: totally normal. If neither of the above: congratulations! Be happy you are so easily aroused and have such an attentive dick. But please also take care that your libidinous zeal doesn't get to be too much for your partner. Your partner's throat may not be quite as robust as your boner. And not every guy is into quickies. Apart from that, ask yourself occasionally, "Oh man, I'm so horny again. Is that normal?" There are two answers to this. The first is another question: What's normal? The second: As long as you can have sex without feeling guilty all the time (whether it's because you've gone overboard, neglected important duties or other areas of your life), there is no cause for concern. But if that happens a lot, you might want to read up on sex addiction. And do something about

it, if necessary. If not, you are in danger of putting too much strain not only on other people but on yourself as well. Especially because you're so robust!
Compatible with: fluffers, gaggers

▼ Jizzers

In your opinion, the main goal is orgasm, and how you get there is a side issue. This pragmatic stance is due either to the fact that you climax relatively quickly, as soon as your dick has passed the ninety degree angle mark, or that you have a fetish for semen. In either case, the "Swallowing" chapter at the end of this book will probably suit your needs. After all, the following pages will focus more on the journey towards orgasm than on what it results in. But perhaps you're here because you've been asking yourself whether your single-minded pursuit of ejaculation might mean you're missing out. It's a legitimate question. The great thing about human (particularly gay) sexuality is that it does not simply serve an instinctively reproductive purpose, but is also something to be enjoyed. It's the same as with food. Instead of just stuffing yourself until you're full, you can savor the taste of your food as well. We will try and expand your capacity for enjoyment in the following chapters. Perhaps you'll take some of it to heart. If not, I can only advise you to inform your sex partners that you're only interested in cumming as quickly as possible—before you go on a date. If you use online dating, put that down in your profile. You'll be able to find men with similar interests more quickly and you will also avoid disappointing your partners.
Compatible with: fluffers, swallowers

> **If you're only interested in cumming as quickly as possible, put that in your profile.**

▼ Fappers

Have you already encountered one or more of the inept blow job providers I mentioned at the beginning of this book? Or do you just not like being in control of what happens to your erection? If one of these descriptions applies to you, you're probably a fapper. Don't get me wrong! I don't mean this offensively. In this context, a fapper is simply the type of man who likes to decide what happens during sex. It doesn't matter whether this is a result of a latent skepticism in your partner's oral skills or of a variety of egotism and self-assurance that can actually be pretty conducive to good sex. The question is simply: How does this affect your actions? It's one thing to just do your own thing, and quite another to give your partner the impression that you would be better off on your own than with him. Of course, there are plenty of submissive tops out there who, in the course of being used, really appreciate the second option, but even then, you should preserve a minimum of empathy. And here's another tip: Perhaps you could try talking to your sex partners some more. Giving up some control over your own boner is a lot easier if you've both agreed on the rules beforehand.
Compatible with: fluffers, swallowers

▼ Explorers

If I compared your dick to the needle on a compass, would you agree? Welcome to the world of explorers. In some ways, this type is a combination of a humpers and a fapper, but he is more consciously aware of his own urges than the former and a lot more open to compromise than the latter. A passionate species, one whose main characteristic is curiosity. Because even though you have gone through all three stages of your genital socialization and the bond between you and your dick has grown closer and more affectionate at every stage, the compass needle between your legs still has the ability to surprise you—an endless fount of new discoveries. If you're not too proud to admit to occasionally not knowing something, you can involve your partner in these explorations. Which is why people never get bored around you. Unless of course, they get sick of discovering new ground. And this is your weak spot: You are fairly demanding. Not necessarily because you have high expectations, but because you expect a lot of dedication from your partner. Because you're able to fully throw yourself into a blow job quickie, you expect your partner to demonstrate a certain degree of dedication. As not everyone can muster up the same sort of enthusiasm all the time—or even wants to—you are easily disappointed. And sometimes offended. Here's a piece of advice for you: Try not to confuse obsessiveness with passion and try to cope with the occasional disappointment without becoming bitter. An impulsive guy like you will sadly meet his share of disappointments. Apart from that, the following chapters should be very enjoyable for you.

Compatible with: gaggers, swallowers, biters

▼ Pashas

When I gave priority to the supported version of lying on your back in our introduction to the basic positions, did you shake your head in disapproval? And was my dismissal of the sideward reclining position even less to your taste? Then you are probably one of the few true pashas, a representative of a species that has grown increasingly rare in today's gay community. Which is to say: A blow job for you consists in lying back on your ottoman and letting your partner do his thing. You don't feel the need to participate actively, nor do you feel under pressure to conform to any kind of performance ideal. What does this have to do with your dick? Presumably the fact that your relationship with your junk is pretty relaxed. It works just fine, but you don't need it distinguish yourself in any way. I congratulate you on your laid-back attitude! Life is there to be enjoyed, like a gentle, clove-scented breeze drifting through your seraglio! But you should be aware that your relaxed attitude may not be enough for many tops. Many of them need a little more impressive behavior from their partners to get in the mood. That may not be your thing but that doesn't mean you can't exploit it for your own purposes from time to time. After all, leaning back and enjoying yourself is a lot more fun if your partner is properly motivated. Apart from that, you're probably more of a relationship kind of guy and don't have

> *Life is there to be enjoyed, like a gentle, clove-scented breeze drifting through your seraglio!*

much time for the whole dating scene, right? That's good. Otherwise you would have to define yourself via your dick. And you probably wouldn't enjoy that as much.
Compatible with: lickers, suckers, biters

▼ Mr. Sensitive

You are very likely not circumcised, you aren't interested in acting the tough guy and you prefer to take things slowly during sex? Then you're probably the type of guy for whom sex is still a very intimate act rather than a public display. This is closely connected with your personal tolerance to sensation. You are very sensitive to touch and your dick in particular is a hallowed area where only a select few may enter. Your partner has to prove he deserves the privilege of being allowed access to your holy of holies. Once he has done so, however, he can be assured of your complete and unfailing dedication. He may even be allowed to handle it a little more firmly. Touch is a matter of trust. This is why monogamy is the only valid relationship form for you. If I had any advice to give you, it would be this: Be true to yourself, but don't make life harder than it needs to be. A date is a date and a blow job is a blow job. Your dick can withstand both of these things and they won't make it any less valuable. The same applies to jerking off.
Compatible with: lickers, suckers

Basic Equipment for Receiving a Blow Job

We have already discussed the demands and limits of your penis, but receiving a blow job involves more than just holding your dick out. The pashas and jizzers among my readers might disagree at first, but if you think about it for a moment, you will agree that the deployment of one or two other limbs and organs may not be mandatory for a good blow job, but it can be helpful. Even if it's just to maintain a pleasant sensation or intensify your climax. So let us take a good look at the libidinous potential of some of the basic equipment that every man owns. Without having to pack a sex-party rucksack or put on a cruising wristband.

▼ Hands

Some things just seem banal until you take a closer look and realize that they are actually pretty complicated. Let's take for example the uncontroversial statement: "Using your hands makes receiving a blow job easier and better." You can stop rolling your eyes: I'm not talking about unzipping your pants, getting your dick out, or giving it a couple of strokes until it's hard. You're obviously going to need your hands for that (unless your partner is especially adept with his lips and teeth). Instead, we're going to take a look at a number of variations on the six "basic holds."

> **The cock ring effect: Place your fingers around the root of your dick and squeeze.**

The holder: You've hauled your dick out of your pants and your partner's mouth is ready and waiting? This is your opportunity for offering your partner a service that will benefit you as well. Make a circle around the root of your dick with your thumb and forefinger, hold your boner directly in front of your partner's face, and squeeze firmly. This will not only leave you in control of the angle and depth, it also produces a kind of cock ring effect. Constricting the root of your penis will make your boner swell up, making it thicker and more sensitive. As always, the general rule here is, don't go overboard and start squeezing too hard. Gentle pressure is enough to produce the cock ring effect, and you will only need to keep it up for a couple of minutes. If you're especially adroit, you can also jam your ball sack between your forefinger and middle finger, just above your nuts, and offer it up for your partner to lick.

The stroker: A blow job always entails having your partner bury his head between your legs. While he's busy down there, you'll have plenty of time to stroke his head, his ears, or the back of his neck. This tender gesture is appreciated by nervous tops in particular, and has its own appeal. Whether the head in your lap is bald or hairy (in which case you can counter the caress by pulling his head back by the hair), sunburned or pale and interesting—there is as much variety in the structure of men's hair and skin as there is in their dicks.

> **A great opportunity to redefine the old saying "His ears were burning."**

The head clamp: If it's going well and your partner is a talented deep-throater, the head clamp is practically a must. Grabbing your partner around the back of his head with both hands and pushing his head down on your boner is a guaranteed kick for everyone involved. While the top gurgles, it's a sensory firework display for the bottom. If your partner is relaxed, you can use only one hand. And if he isn't fussy, you can grab hold of his ears and use those as handles. A nice opportunity for redefining the old saying "His ears were burning."

The choker: Please take extra special care for this one! Placing your hands around the bottom's throat, controlling his movements and, if that's your thing, choking him a little clearly requires a lot of trust. This is definitely not first-date material, nor should you

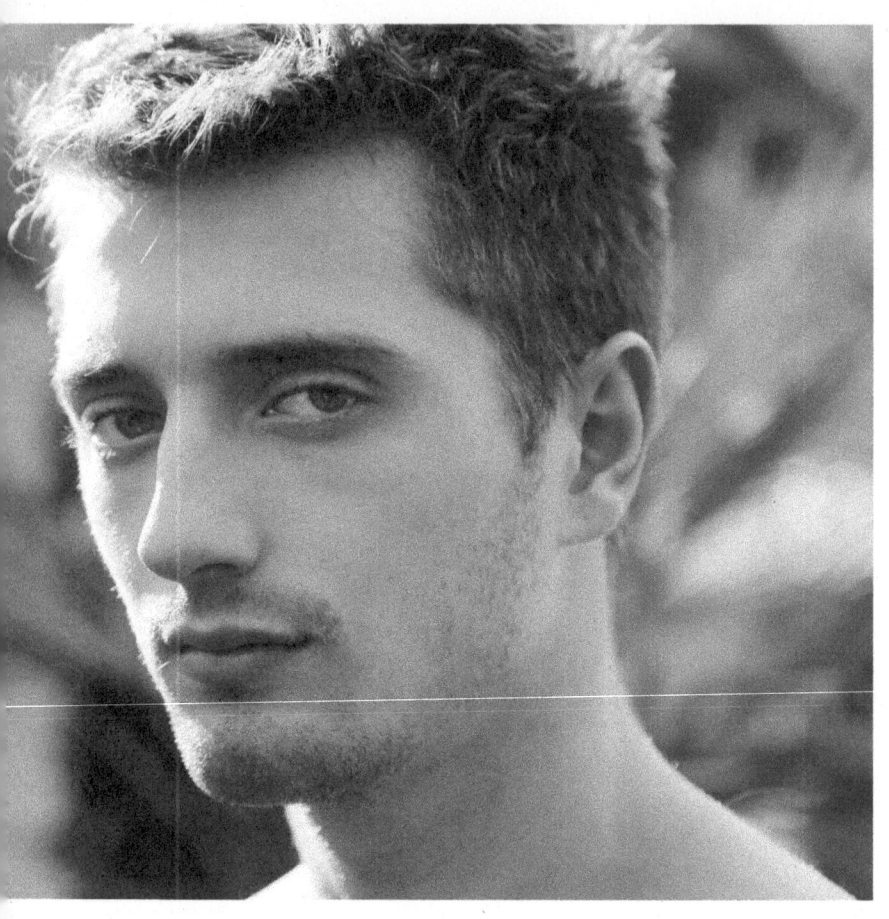

spring it on your partner without warning or prior discussion. But as many tops find it a real turn on, it makes no sense not to mention it here, at the very least.

The groper: This term says everything and nothing. As a bottom doesn't actually need to use his hands at all, these can be employed for specific moves or just for general groping purposes. In some ways, this is an extended version of the stroker. You can let your hands wander down your partner's shoulders and back to his ass, or you can selfishly use them to stimulate your own nipples, hips, or ass crack. What you do with them generally depends on your partner. You should always try groping your partner to see if he enjoys it. Some guys find it extremely motivating.

▼ Eyes

Closing your eyes and concentrating entirely on the sensual input while you're receiving a blow job can be very stimulating, but we will go into that later. For the reverse is also true: Looking can be a strong emotional catalyst as well. Whether you're just enjoying the pornographic view of the top toiling over your dick or trying to maintain eye contact with him, your eyes can help enhance your pleasure. Besides which, you can always use them to guide the action. Sometimes an encouragingly raised eyebrow can say much more than a crude "Go on, deeper," and a pleading face is frequently a more direct expression of arousal than a run of the mill moan. Proper moaning is an entire science in its own right, but we'll go into that presently. Let me point just one thing out: Plenty of blow job tops tend to be pretty shy and even slightly ashamed of what they're doing. An unmistakable sign of this is if they consistently avoid looking up. Insisting on eye contact can help them overcome their inhibitions. You can even turn this into a game by constantly reminding your partner to look up at you while he's busy—even if this runs the risk of distracting him from his oral endeavors and putting him off his stroke.

▼ Ball Sack

Grabbing your balls between your fingers in the "holder" position to draw your lover's attention to them is, of course, not the only way you can incorporate them into a blow job. You can do this more systematically by asking your partner for an explicit ball-licking intermezzo. Nut fetishists are aware that this is often necessary, as many blow job artists are so fixated on dicks, they tend forget about anything else. Which leads us straight to the ambivalence surrounding "tea bagging" (sucking a man's balls). The problem here is, not many people have much experience with this. Which inevitably leads to you having to help them out to prevent damage to your crown jewels. A clumsy ball licker can cause a lot more pain than an inexperienced blow job artist. To prevent accidents, it's best to proceed systematically.

Point 1 – Ask yourself: Am I into ball play? By which I mean, do you intuitively involve your balls while you're having sex or jerking off? If that is the case, you can move on to the next point, as you are already well aware of your ball sack's hotspots and no-go areas. If you haven't paid much attention to your nuts up till now, fiddle with them a bit first. You might discover a new erogenous zone. First steps include massaging, stroking, and gently tugging your scrotum. Lube, ball rings, shaved pube,s or structured utensils (brushes, knobs, smooth surfaces) can help you explore your own preferences. After that, you should be sufficiently sensitized and aware of how much your balls can take to surrender them up to your blow job partners (or to withhold them, if it turns out not to be your thing).

Point 2 – Be demanding: If your date doesn't pay attention to your family jewels of his own accord, let him know. Either by shoving them into his mouth or by telling him to "Lick my balls."

Point 3 – Try it out: As I said before, many blow job tops will not have much experience with balls or not know what to do with them. You'll know soon enough whether your partner is one of those guys. Wild, uncoordinated licking or rough sucking are generally unmistakable signs. But they are no reason to reject ball-sucking out of hand. Just move on to point 4.

Point 4 – The workshop: Sometimes you have to approach sex didactically if you want to increase the pleasure on both sides. In the highly individualized case of customizing your own nut-pam-

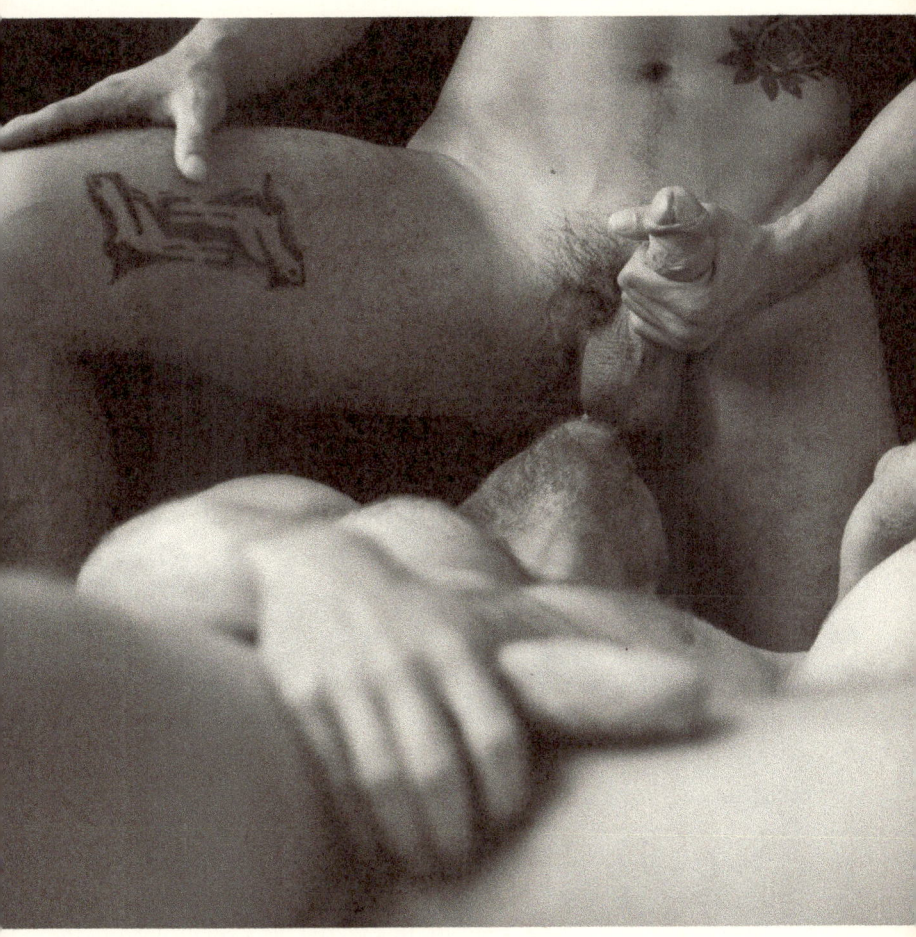

pering program, this is generally unavoidable. By which I mean, show your lover what you want! In principle, all you have to do is repeat your previous self-exploratory sessions with your partner. Tugging, massaging, pulling the skin of your sack tight. All of this can be undertaken by your partner, as long as you show him what to do. Besides which, his tongue is a beautifully structured tool. Keep polishing those family jewels!

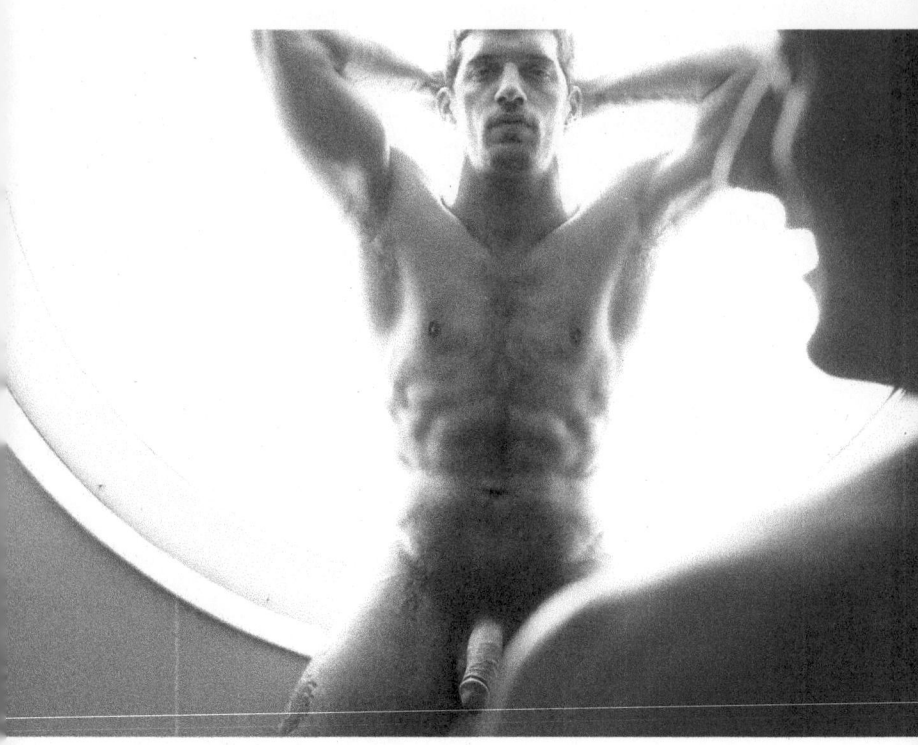

▼ Hips

There's a gay myth that suggests that watching a guy dance will tell you everything you need to know about his qualities in bed. I have never been able to confirm this myself, as a sexy swing of the hips on the dancefloor does not always translate to fun in the sack, but that doesn't mean there's no truth in the statement "My hips don't lie." If you are relaxed and rhythmic, you are probably quite in tune with your body, which makes it easier to use it consciously during sex. What has this got to do with blow jobs? It's quite simple: *Move your hips, baby!* Moving your hips to enhance a blow job is an expression of skill and creativity. There are a number of basic techniques that can be varied at will. Here they are!

The pelvic thrust: Meet your partner halfway during a blow job to do justice to the term "mouth fucking." Which is one excellent reason for doing it. The basic principle is to thrust your hips backwards and forwards to regulate the depth of penetration. Proceed carefully, as this requires a lot of practice on both sides.

The lapdance: Mix it up! Instead of moving his head and tongue to increase the stimulation, ask your top to hold still for a while. Have him take as much of your boner as possible into his mouth and let you regulate the stimulation by circling your hips. You can even use a corkscrew motion to penetrate deeper. This technique does require a certain amount of talent on the part of the top to be really enjoyable. Other possible, but less popular alternatives include moving from side to side or up and down.

The freestyler: A really hot activity for your breaks is to rub or thrust your saliva-lubed dick in your partner's face after a couple of rounds of deep-throating by moving your hips around (without touching it with your hands).

▼ Voice

As the previously discussed points on asking your partner to lick your balls or maintaining eye contact have shown, communication is an important part of sex. In fact, sex is an act of communication in itself. So you shouldn't be afraid to talk during a blow job. Especially as the top's mouth will frequently be too full to be able to speak up for himself. Spur him on and keep up the

> *If you want to do justice to the term "mouth fuck," you'll have to meet your partner halfway.*

connection between the two of you by checking up on him from time to time. Ask him if he likes it. Does he want more? Has he always been such a hot mouth slut? And so on. The smothered "mm-mmm" responses to your questions will be enough to make them worth your while. This takes us to the more abstract uses of the human voice. You can use your own to make other sounds apart from actual speech. You can easily spice up a hot session by, instead of just receiving the blow job in stony silence, gasping, breathing heavily or purring with contentment to let your partner know how aroused you are.

▼ Ass

Many blow job bottoms identify as tops on a fundamental level, which frequently gets in the way of their enjoying any anal benefits. But this is not an impediment, just another reason for going into this topic in more detail at this point. While the chapter on "Rimming" on page 160 deals explicitly with the topic of eating ass, we will take a look at some of the preliminary steps here. Because you can of course extend your auto-groping endeavors to include using your hands to massage and open up your anus. You can also ask your partner, in addition or as an alternative to sucking your balls, to provide you with an anal finger job. Another really sexy option: Show up for your blow job date with a butt plug in your anus, and ask your partner to tap the base while he sucks you off. Or do it yourself. All of these methods are a bonus program to supplement your genital stimulation. They also offer the bottom the opportunity of adding a certain degree of ambiguity to his own role. A manly blow job bottom with a plug in his ass creates the tantalizing suggestion that he might also be open to bottoming during anal sex, an idea that many men will find incredibly erotic. Meanwhile the guy wearing the plug gets to enjoy high-quality stimulation from both sides. It's a win-win situation!

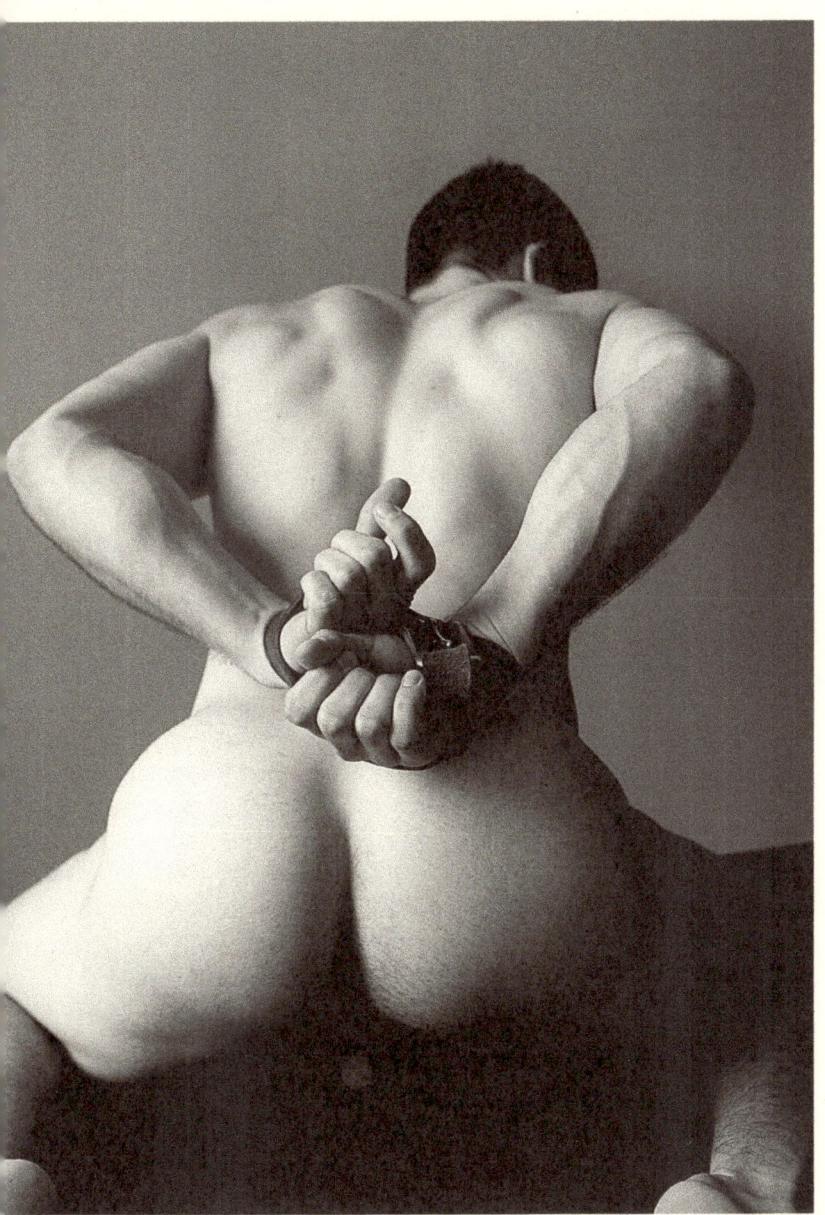

Blow Job Boot Camp for Bottoms

While there are plenty of practical exercises for tops who want to train their blow job skills, there are also many ways in which a bottom can prepare himself for a blow job—physically, intellectually, and mentally. And there are good reasons for doing so. It's easier to surrender yourself up, close your eyes, and enjoy if you know what you're doing and what you want. Especially because if you do encounter a situation that isn't going according to plan, you'll have a better chance of identifying the root of the problem and finding a solution. The purpose of the following seven exercises is to make you more consciously aware of the blow job bottom's most important tool: his tool. What gets it up? What brings it down? And what role do other parts of your body play in either event? If you can answer these questions, you can communicate clearly with your partner, which will have an effect on the length and intensity of your encounter. The other purpose of these exercises is of course to make a ridiculous amount of mess, break down any preconceived notions and embark on a program of instructive silliness. Clean-freaks (put down a waterproof liner or some garbage bags beforehand) and stressed out practitioners of purely functional masturbation (block at least two hours in your diary and label them as "fun") will have a hard time with these exercises. We are here to have fun. Because that's what oral sex should be about.

> **Block at least two hours in your diary for "fun" and "mess."**

Most of you will need to take a break in between exercises; nevertheless, try and have all the items on your shopping list on page 113 to hand, just in case. Your melon should be stored at room temperature, not refrigerated. Concerning the glasses, aim for a range of sizes. As you will probably have guessed, you will be sticking your dick into them, so the diameter of the opening should be larger than that of your erect penis. Anything else should become clear later on. But now, it's on your marks, get set, go! We'll start out with a simple, almost meditative exercise.

▼ Exercise 1: The Feather

A word in advance: The feathers employed in this exercise should not be teeny tiny down feathers or fluffy marabou feathers. They should produce a certain degree of resistance. Goose feathers (the kind that used to serve as writing quills) are a good choice. You can also use an old-fashioned feather duster if you own such a thing. How to proceed: Take off your clothes, relax, think happy thoughts, or watch a porn movie and masturbate until you're hard. Getting it up is part of preparatory stage. Once it's up, literally screen yourself off from visual stimuli. So if you've been watching a porn movie, turn off your computer or DVD—and put that magazine away! Now it's just you and your boner. And the feathers, of course. Pick these up and use them to stroke the tip and the shaft of your penis—and don't forget your balls. The amount of pressure you exert will depend on the general and current tolerance of your dick. Some of you will hardly feel anything at all and be thinking "What's the fucking point of this?" while others will feel a shudder coursing through their bodies, giving them goosebumps and stiffening their nipples. Neither of these reactions is better than the other one. Because from this point on, I'd like you to explore.

> *Some will say, "What's the fucking point of this?" while others feel their nipples getting hard.*

If you can't feel anything, find the ticklish spots. If you can barely stand it, find a way to keep going without losing your erection. And take your time! When you're done, you'll have an approximate idea of where the hot-spots on your boner are, which will later become attractive points for targeted licking. This exercise is also a great test of stamina for your erection. By the way, if the feathers are just too soft for you (although this is largely a question of attitude), you can use a more solid object such as a spoon or a teabag (these aren't bad), or if you're extremely robust, try using the fibers (or even the handle) of a soft toothbrush. As long

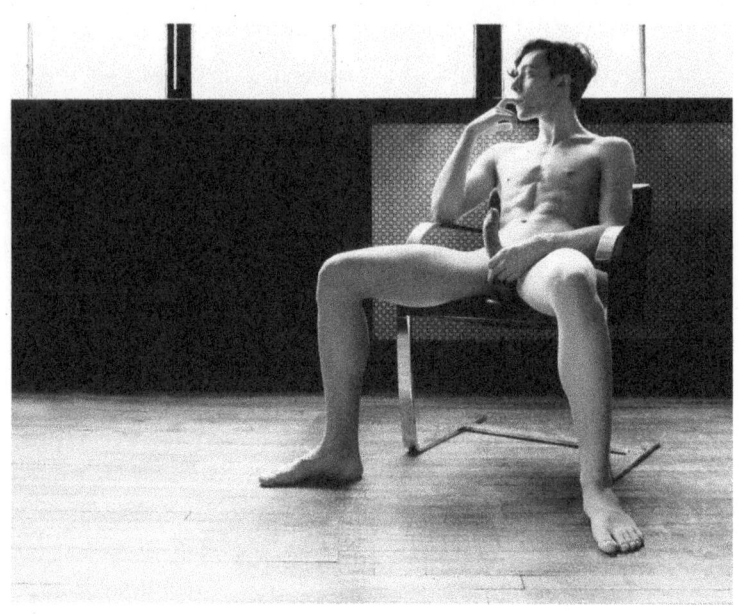

as it makes you tingle. Without using lube. We'll take a closer look at lubes in a minute. Apart from that, try not to cum! You need to keep your head switched on to find your hot spots. If you're forgetful, write them down on a piece of paper and place it next to your bed. The next time you masturbate, you can use this as a roadmap to activate your sensitive spots—or give it to your partner to consult during your next blow job date.

▼ Exercise 2: Wet Dreams

I recommend embarking on this exercise immediately after the first, without taking a break. Why? Because now you're going to lube up your boner and gradually increase the intensity, starting at the point you reached during the previous exercise. Once you think you've identified your personal stimulus points with the feather, spit into your hand and spread the saliva over your boner. You will have to repeat this several times and depending on the consistency of your saliva, you might have to switch to lube at some point. But the main goal is a dripping wet dong. Some of you will probably be thinking, "Yuck, this is gross, what is this filthy-minded weirdo up to?" But I'm serious. This time, I want you to go completely overboard! Make it really sticky and wet. If you're worried about the rug, put something waterproof on top first. You've already invested in plenty of paper towels, just in case. There are three reasons it needs to be this wet.

First: to get you accustomed to the drooling and dribbling, which for some blow job artists constitutes the main attraction.
Secondly: It will make your dick nice and slippery and less sensitive to touch.
Thirdly: It will help you get over your feelings of disgust, feelings that should generally be screened out during sexual activities as they can present a serious barrier to your pleasure. There are even academic studies that show that during sex, certain parts of the brain that normally process triggers for disgust are switched off. This dampens your reluctance to expose yourself or your mucous membranes to certain body fluids in favor of sheer animal lust— and animal lust is a great aspect of sex. When you're masturbating, which is what the "Wet Dreams" exercise is ultimately about, you have to compensate for the lack of erotic stimulus, the touch and smell of your lover, by mobilizing these "switching off" mechanisms yourself. Which is what makes this a good exercise for lowering your tolerance threshold for physical contact with your partner. And for some people, it's also a way to increase their acceptance of their bodies and bodily fluids.

The rest is a matter of applying lube, applying more lube, and then jerking off some more. Try placing one fist on top of the other to simulate a mouth around your dick. And make sure you don't forget the glans. It's a good idea to desensitize this part of your body beforehand. Apart from that, try to delay your orgasm for as long as possible. This will increase your stamina. But once you do reach the point of ejaculation, you've definitely earned it.

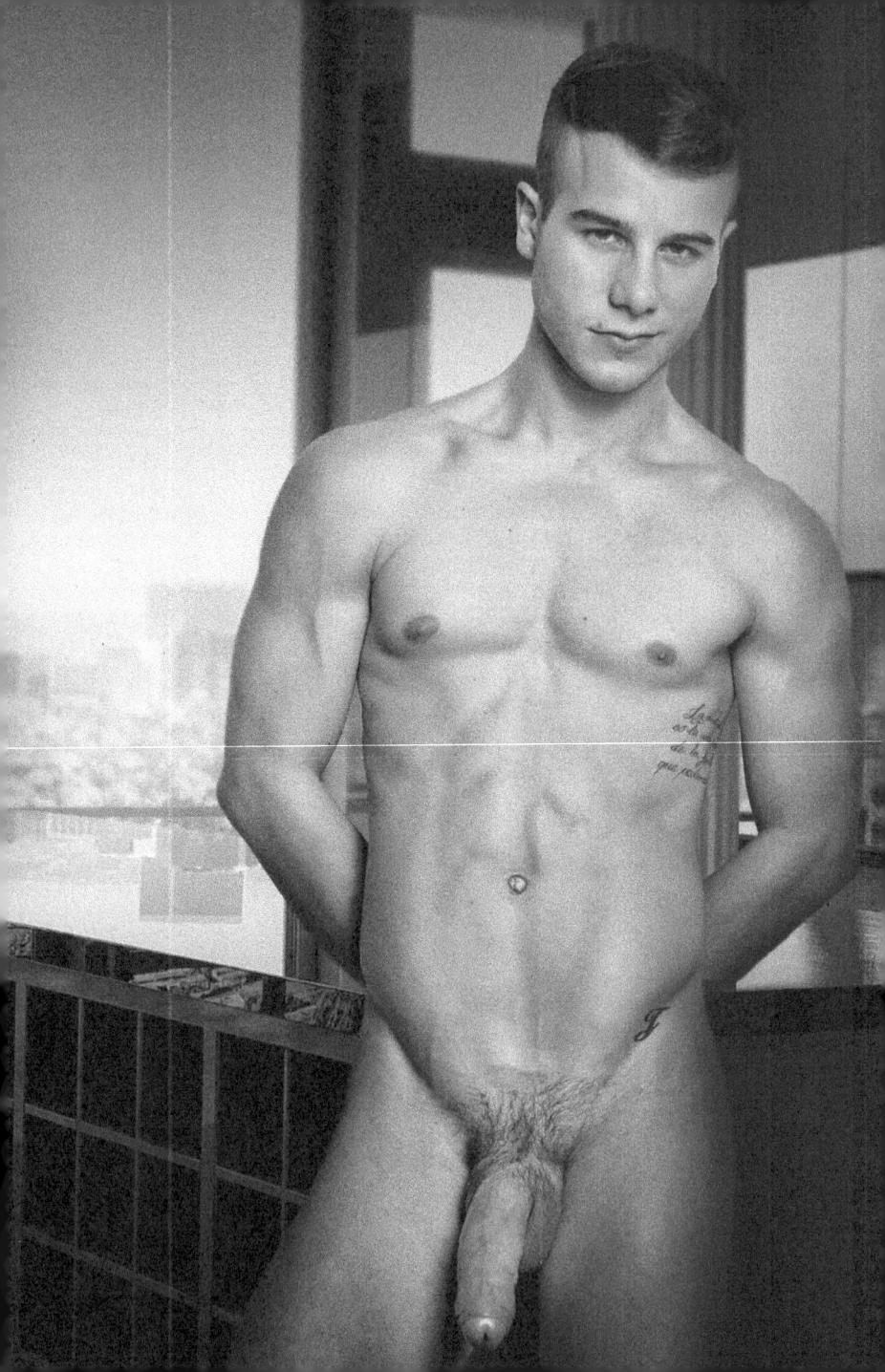

▼ Exercise 3: The Melon

Those of my readers who are already familiar with my *Gayma Sutra* will know what to expect at this point. This book included a section entitled "Masturbation Positions," one of which was called "Fucking A Melon." At the time, I introduced this position as follows: "Cutting a hole in a melon, digging yourself a fuck-channel and then—I beg you!—first putting a condom on your dick and sticking it in is above all an unholy mess." I have nothing to add to this. For even after having seduced a wide range of fruit and vegetables (admittedly, for the first time since researching the *Gayma Sutra*), I can confirm that the sticky mess this involved definitely overstepped the boundaries of what is generally considered acceptable. Fortunately, I had just graduated from the "Wet Dreams" program for blocking out feelings of disgust and general ickiness. The reason I still think a melon is a great tool for practicing on is because it does give you the feeling of pushing a man's head (even though melons are a lot heavier, smoother and rounder than your average head) down onto your dick. Depending on how narrow you've made it, the edges of the fuck channel do a pretty good job of simulating the boundaries you're boner will come up against inside your partner's mouth. I suggest you make the channel slightly wider, rather than too tight. Otherwise it will be uncomfortable and you will end up squeezing tons of pulp and juice out of the opening with your boner, and it will all run down your leg. Apart from that, make sure the melon isn't too cold, otherwise you can say goodbye to your erection. Please do not try to warm it up in the microwave! It will get too hot and go all squishy. You can stick it in the oven briefly and let it cool off, but the best thing is to leave it out at room temperature overnight—before cutting a hole into it. Always cut the hole just before you start fucking the melon. The benefits of this exercise for oral sex are also explained in *Gayma Sutra*, where I have also provided a blow job version of the same (replacing the melon with another man's head) entitled "Melonhead."

▼ Exercise 4: Fucking a Glass

Once you've recovered from your exertions with the melon and had a good wash, we'll turn our attention to the glasses. The point of this exercise is to force your dick into contact with a resisting surface while at the same time, giving you a visual illustration of what happens inside your partner's mouth while he's sucking you off. Grab a champagne glass, lube up your boner, and stick it in. Depending on the length of your cock, the head will probably hit the bottom of the glass. This is the point we're aiming for. Because it will help you realize that gentle pressure on your glans is not in itself painful. Your dick is tough enough to deal with any bottleneck situation it is likely to encounter in your partner's mouth. If the glass is too large, pick a shorter or smaller one or you could even try sticking your glans into a thimble-sized glass (such as a shot glass). Please don't squash it! Squeezing your precious manhood into a too-small tube or orifice is not the point of this exercise. Instead, make sure there is always just a little wiggle room around the sides. You should only encounter resistance when you reach the bottom—you don't want to get stuck. Funnel-shaped glasses that open up at the top are the best choice. Avoid using very thin glasses that might break. One more tip: If you find the sensation of glass on your dick unpleasant, put a condom on beforehand. That helps.

> *Glans meets glass—a taste of bottlenecks to come.*

If you've fulfilled all these requirements, you are now in a position to fully enjoy the visual and sensual benefits of fucking a glass. Rub your lubed-up shaft against the inside of the glass, test your tolerance by gently bumping the tip against the bottom of the glass, try out different shapes and sizes. Once you've felt and seen enough, move on to the Cocktail Test. Fill the glasses with liquid (carbonated/uncarbonated, viscous/watery) or mush, place them on the ground and dip your wick into them from a push-up position. You can feel the difference between different substances and it is also good preparation for any games with your partner involving food.

▼ **Exercise 5: Fangs**

A top's teeth are a bottom's worst enemy. If your partner is unable to keep them under control, the results can be very unpleasant. To prepare yourself for the worst case scenario, you're going to need one of those crappy sets of plastic fangs commonly sold to children (and adults) around Halloween, when everyone parades around in their Dracula/*Twilight*-themed costumes. These plastic snappers are rarely any good and tend to slip out at the slightest provocation, but they are perfect for our purposes. Depending on the girth and sensitivity of your dick, you can always file them down. If you do this, make sure you don't produce any rough edges that might scrape your dick. Although... Ultimately, that's what this exercise is about. Hold the fangs between the thumbs and forefingers of both hands, turn them so that they are facing your boner, and then carefully place then over the glans—leaving your dick caught between the "jaws." Then move the fangs carefully up and down your shaft. Tough guys won't need lube, everyone else might want to apply a little beforehand. Gradually change the pressure on your dick, again with care and concentration. It will feel bizarre, unfamiliar and not particularly pleasant at first, but after a while, a few of you might notice that certain types of pressure do in fact feel quite nice. Or that there's something to be said for a gentle "bite" around the root of your dick. Or that after messing around for a bit, using the fangs to play with your glans, balls, or nipples suddenly seems like a good idea. In the latter scenario, you might find yourself on the brink of a full-fledged biting fetish, so do inform your partner of this before your next date. If not, you now know what it feels like to have teeth scraping along your boner—and identifying and, if necessary, curtailing the actions of a "bitey" top will be a lot easier.

▼ **Exercise 6: Blind Faith**

Time to take stock! If you think back to the previous five exercises, you should ideally have enjoyed all of them, but most people will have developed specific preferences. If you enjoyed the fangs, you

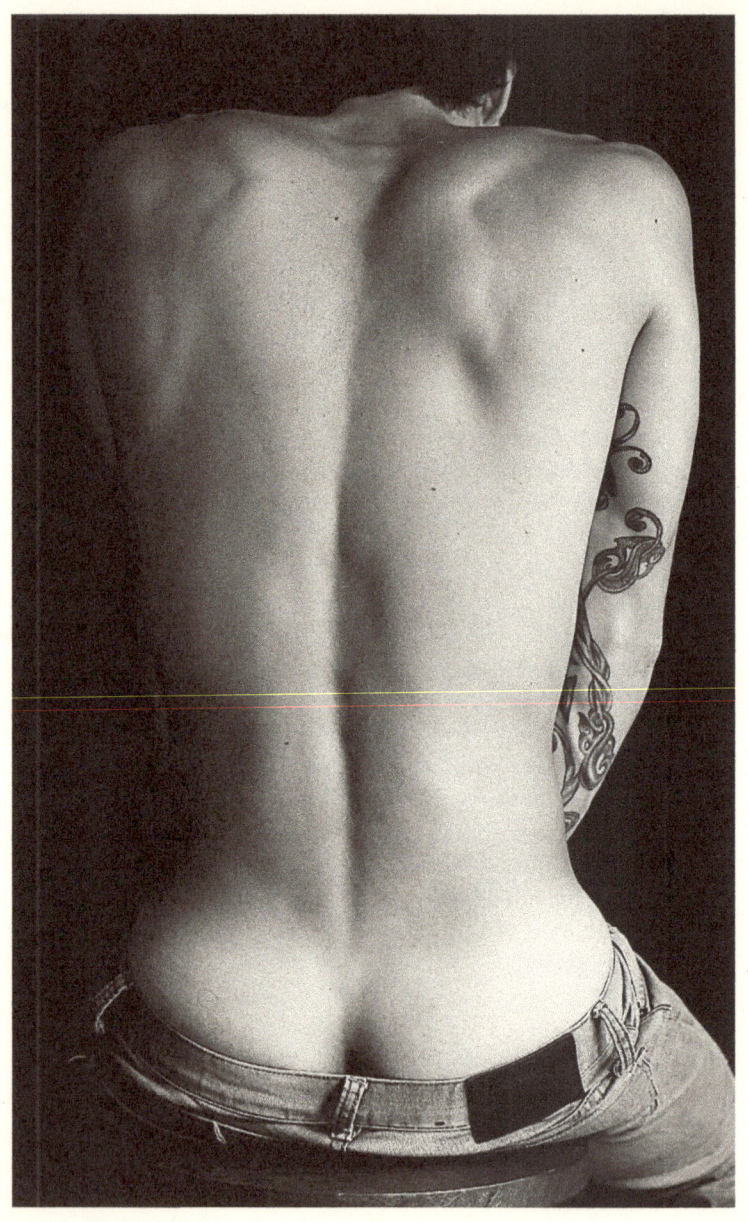

were probably bored to distraction by the feathers. If the hot mess of melons and "Wet Dreams" was exciting, the fangs were probably the opposite. Either way, we are now going to intensify our experience by repeating our favorite exercises, this time while wearing a blindfold. This will further enhance your sensitivity to weak spots and hot spots and force you to take everything just a little more slowly. Both of which contributes to the fine

> *Once the blindfold's in place, you'll have finally "Shut Your Eyes."*

tuning of your erotic sensors, which is the main goal of this boot camp. In some ways, it also intensifies the feeling of being alone with your dick produced in exercise one by setting aside all visual (pornographic) aids. Thanks to the blindfold, you are not only alone with your boner, you are also robbed of your sight and have finally reached the "Shut Your Eyes" mode announced at the beginning of this section. Everything else is a matter of exploring by touch, being aware of your own reactions and, once you've overcome any initial coordination issues, pleasure.

▼ Exercise 7: Masturbator Action

Once you've fucked a melon and a wide array of glassware, you have probably realized that you can stick your dick into practically anything if you're motivated enough. These exercises are also a simple and inexpensive method of testing the boundaries of your own erectile temperament. This is, of course, a lot easier if you have a device that has been explicitly designed for this purpose. There are quite a number of these on the market. So if you would like to continue to improve your skills using more professional equipment, turn the page for an overview of the wonderful world of masturbators.

FIVE MASTURBATOR TYPES

▼ 1 – Blow Job Machine

No article on masturbators would be complete without mentioning the phenomenon of blow job machines, but as I've already gone into them in great detail on pages 31 to 33, I would refer anyone interested in these devices to those pages. I would just like to add that using a vacuum cleaner or other household appliance to make your own is inadvisable. For one thing, most of them don't work, and for another, the risk of injuring yourself is greater than any potential pleasure factor.

▼ 2 – Fleshjacks

Fleshjacks derive their name from their shape, which is similar to that of a large flashlight. The part of the flashlight where the light comes out is the part of the Fleshjack where something goes in: your dick. You can choose from a number of differently shaped openings: mouth, vagina, or miniature butt, all made from elastic cyberskin rubber, which is flexible enough to accommodate even the most well-endowed and firm enough to create resistance. As long as you use enough lube, you can fuck these things until you're tired. To clean your Fleshjack, remove the fuck tube from its hard plastic casing, turn it inside out, and put it back in place once it's dried. In brief, this is a masturbatory aid that can be used any number of times and, while it cannot take the place of a real blow job, does provide you with a surprisingly good imitation. You can also order a variety of structured linings for the fuck tube as well as choose from a range of (ostensibly) realistic replicas of porn stars' mouths and anuses, among them Cockyboy Jake Bass, who is featured on page 95 of this book.

▼ 3 – Pocket Pussy

These are available from condom vending machines and in some drugstores. They closely resemble an inflatable plastic bag which, when inflated, turns into a ring-shaped air cushion. You insert your lubed-up dick into the middle of the ring and move it (the ring or your boner, according to preference) up and down. Despite the astoundingly simple principle involved and the incredibly cheap execution, these things fulfill their purpose surprisingly well. I would not, however, recommend reusing them.

▼ 4 – Sex Doll

Not a recommendation, but it is a possibility. If you've got money to burn or enjoy feeling ridiculous during solo oral sex, you can treat yourself to a sex doll. There is a far larger variety of female dolls, complete with perfectly spherical breasts and three holes (mouth-anus-vajayjay) on the market, but you can get male versions, too (often featuring a vibrating dong). Using one of these to practice for the real thing is both ridiculous and grotesque. But so is sex with a real partner—at least sometimes. This is, however, the only realistic aspect of these dolls.

▼ 5 – Pumps

Vacuum pumps to pump up your dick (which is why they are also used to treat erectile dysfunction) are fine for experimenting with and can contribute to you getting up just a little more substance to fill your partner's mouth with. But the sensations resulting from pumping have nothing in common with how your dick feels inside another man's mouth. There simply isn't enough friction.

Get That Fuck Mouth—How to Do it!

It can't be avoided. At some point, you're going to have to tear yourself away from your beloved melons and masturbators and set out into the wide world of men—who are, after all, the reason we started fostering friendships between fruit, glasses, upcycled flashlights, and our genitals in the first place. It would be a pity to make them wait any longer. After all, there are thousands of gay men out there waiting eagerly for a new dick to suck—and one of them may be waiting for yours in particular. But there's plenty of time for romance later. For the present, I am here to tell you the following: As a stalwart blow job bottom (once you've graduated from our boot camp), you stand a pretty good chance of encountering a mass of hungry mouths. But be aware: They are demanding, they can sometimes be impatient, and in their insatiable hunger for dick, they are often merciless. I know, this sounds a bit over the top, but I'm completely serious. Self-avowed mouth sluts tend to fixate on a particular type (not to mention particular size and girth) of dick, and can get very unpleasant if you don't live up to their expectations.

You don't need to let yourself be intimidated or annoyed by this behavior as long as you are honest and realistic about your own qualities. To do this, you've already identified your dick type. And you've tested your sensitivity with a feather. And checked out your tolerance thresholds with a glass. And so on. Everyone will have run into trouble with one of the previous exercises or another and everyone will have gotten tired of the entire thing at some point. That's perfectly normal and even necessary. Remember what parts put you off your stroke so that you can avoid them during actual oral sex. On the other hand, think back to those parts you enjoyed the most, or turned you on the most, as well. You should communicate these to your partners. For example, by adding them to your dating profile. Which takes us to the first of four strategies for meeting, exploring, and hopefully conquering the world of men.

▼ Blow Job Dating

We're talking about online dating here, which is without question the simplest, most practical, and in many aspects most effective way of finding sexually compatible men. I'm not sure I need to tell you this, but here goes: Even though we used the term "bottom" to refer to the person receiving the blow job throughout the course of this chapter, you should not use it in your profile or any of your texts. It is open to misconception. Instead, you could right something like "I love receiving oral" or "Would like to meet a real mouth slut" or similar, so the other guys know what they're dealing with. Returning to the merciless mouth sluts: Please do not try to improve your chances by lying about your dick size. If you make unfounded XXL claims, you will first get yourself into trouble with size queens who have picked you just because of these claims, and second, you won't get the chance to meet people who are actually your size. Cheating in any respect isn't a great idea. Furthermore, once you've set up a date, make sure you turn up on time and are freshly washed and ready for action. Keep your profile pictures updated—add the respective dates to let people know what you currently look like. And read through all the Do's and Don'ts listed on page 146 / 147 beforehand.

▼ Blow Job Cruising

Darkrooms, saunas, adult movie theaters, cruising parks, and highway rest areas—these have always been locations for gay men looking for, and generally finding, sexual contact. The general system of "What you see is what you get" makes cheating impossible, preferences are communicated via posing, glances, or even the handkerchief code. (A light blue bandana in your left back pocket is commonly taken to mean "blow job bottom." The left side is generally the top side—although again, the designations are somewhat open to misunderstandings). Of course, this can be quickly cleared up when you're face to face. Again, pay attention to your personal hygiene and don't be too pushy. If you can't get it up, take a break. Otherwise it's just going to get really unsexy for everyone involved. In general, a clean, hard dick will rarely have long to wait for a hungry mouth.

▼ Blow Job Relationships

It's similar to the fuck buddy principle, just applied to the realm of the blow job. It's no different to a blow job relationship. An excellent model! It's a sure guarantee of familiarity, certainty, and satisfaction. As chemistry and shared appeal play an important part here, you can't force it, but if you are attentive enough to realize that a sex date or cruising encounter has led to a high degree of mutual satisfaction, a simple "Why don't we do this again sometime?" may result in a long and happy blow job relationship. This may also lead to a more exclusive type of relationship, but that isn't the main point of this model.

▼ Blow Job Orgies

If you browse through the dating forums, you'll find a club for every preference, and if you like having your dick sucked by an entire group of men, tags such as "bukkake," "sex party," or simply "orgy" will lead you straight to what you want. Or you could always start your own group. You should, however, be aware that, in most cases, these groups don't stop at the relatively "soft" oral category and generally involve anal sex as well. If this isn't your thing, for whatever reason, don't feel pressured to comply. But you will have to accept the fact that you simply aren't part of the target group for some of these parties.

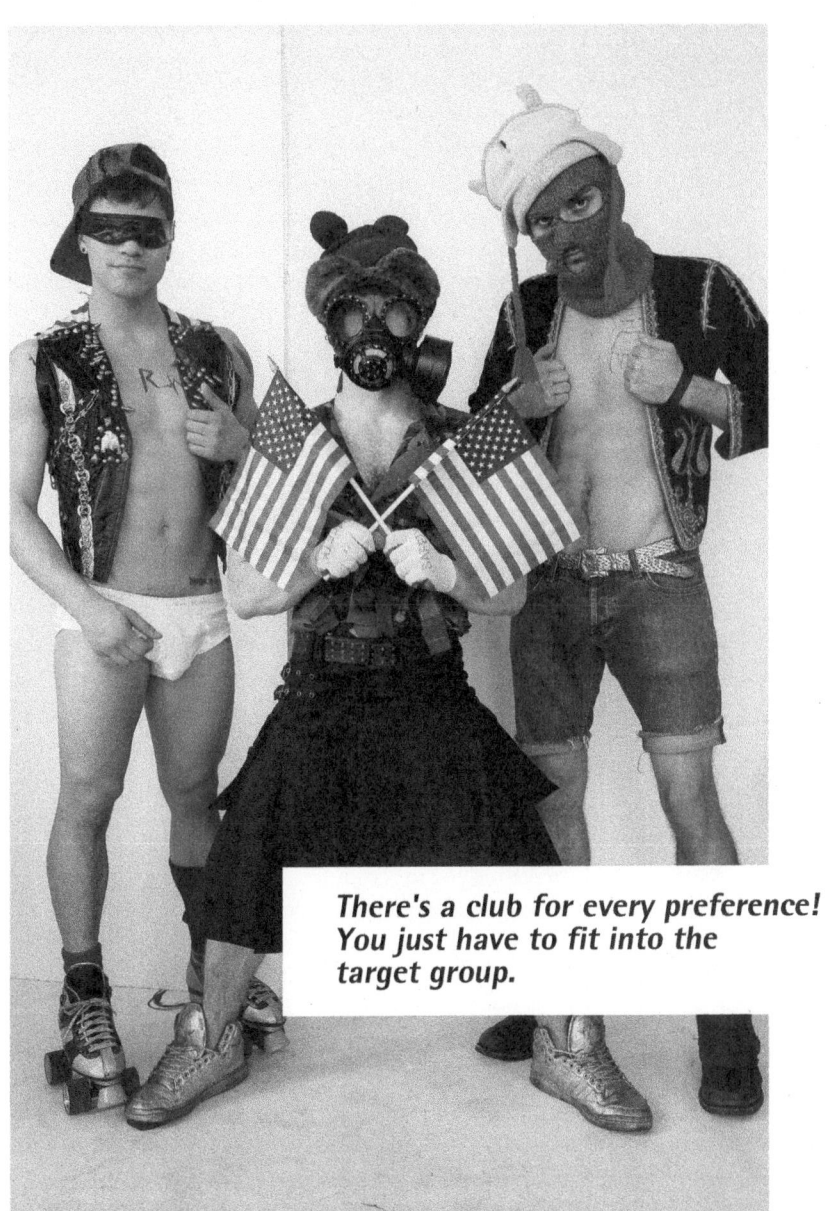

There's a club for every preference! You just have to fit into the target group.

Do's When Receiving a Blow Job

1 - Praise
Compliments will motivate even the most average blow job artist to aspire to higher things. The careful use of praise can serve your interests as well. You don't need to praise him for skills he doesn't actually have, but you can encourage him by showing your appreciation of his strengths, rather than demoralize him with constant criticism.

2 - Specialties
If you can come up with original ideas that aren't part of the standard program, you are sure to inspire both respect and loyalty in your blow job buddy. A signature style will lend you a cachet of individuality among the mass of competitors. What type of style depends on the type of person. This can be anything, from memorable moves to elaborate penile decorations.

3 - Authority
No, there's no need to reveal your inner macho, but you should be aware of his presence inside of you. This means knowing what you want and what you like. Coming up against an indecisive dick is an extremely tedious and unedifying experience for a top. Besides, some people like a bit of machismo from time to time.

4 - Open-mindedness
As your function during the proceedings (holding out your dick) can get a little monotonous, it's important to be open to variety. Keep an open mind to your partner's suggestions. And if their suggestions involve getting a second or even a third dick to join you, try and see it as a challenge rather than a threat.

5 - Returning the Favor
You've cum and now you're all set to leave? Some blow job tops like it that way, but if they want to cum themselves, you should have the decency to return the favor. By sucking or jerking them off, or just by sticking around until they've cum themselves. Now you're even!

Don'ts When Receiving a Blow Job

1 – Uncleanliness
Sure, some tops are into dick cheese and funky pubes, but they tend to communicate this preference beforehand. The rest should be presented with a clean and hygienic dick, if only for health reasons. That doesn't mean you have to shave off your pubes (although that is the most hygienic option), but you should certainly wash them beforehand.

2 – Coercion
Let me be perfectly clear here: Anything you have to use force to achieve is an absolute no-no. Even if you and your partner have agreed that you can get a little rough with him. Coercion means insisting on a specific act that the top has already refused to do. It simply isn't fair to put pressure on him.

3 – Stress
The point of this Don't is to take the pressure off you as well. If it isn't fair to put pressure on your partner, you shouldn't do it to yourself, either. This means, if you're distracted or having trouble getting it up, spare yourself and your partner the tedium of constant stopping, frenetic rubbing, and restarting. That isn't much fun for either of you.

4 – Dismissiveness and Neglect
As a blow job bottom, you have certain responsibilities. It's fine to let yourself be serviced, but you still have to respond to your partners' needs as well. But first, you have to be aware of their needs. So pay attention. For more information, check out the "Fapper" section under "Dick Types."

5 – Ejaculating Without Prior Warning
The timely utterance of the words "I'm about to cum" is not just a matter of safer sex. You should also give your partner the opportunity of either sharing the orgasm he has worked so hard on or taking cover.

The Triumph of Technique: Blow Job Methods for Bottoms

▼ The Switch

Power play forms part of the background of every blow job. But you can also make it part of the foreground. Tell your lover to sit up and beg like a dog. Or tie him up. Either way, he needs to sit still for you to give him a taste of the switch. Getting your flaccid penis out and using it to whip your partner's face, neck, shoulders, and forehead can be great fun. As soon as you have a hard-on, your lover needs to beg for it. Whether or not you let him have it depends on whether he's a good boy. Otherwise, it's time for another taste of the switch. Only do this if your partner enjoys being submissive.

▼ Live Contest

For this method, you will need a webcam, a gay video-chat account, an exhibitionistic streak, and an ambitious partner. You can use these ingredients to transform your domestic blow job into a live show and your sexual pleasure into a competition for the favor of your audience. Some tops outdo themselves under these conditions. You might as well. But you need to discuss whether your public performance will have any negative effects on either of you. If so, you should both wear a mask.

▼ Unwrapping

Nibbling a semi-hard dick through the fabric of your underpants until it's hard and damp is one of the best kinds of foreplay there is. You can systematically delay the final unwrapping and presentation of your naked boner in all its glory. This gives it more significance. And it also contributes to your awareness of the power of your own manhood over your partner. Certain types of outfit or fabric can contribute to this. Short nylon shorts are great, as are not-too-tight bathing trunks, or even a pair of beer-soaked tighty whities.

▼ Extended Play

If you're in a stable blow job relationship or a very open one, you can involve a third man to reach new heights of oral pleasure. Trying to stuff your own dick and that of a fellow bottom into your top's mouth is a great option. Or you could find a trainee top to join your partner as they both get to work on your boner. In either case, everyone involved must agree to it beforehand, and no one should feel neglected or overwhelmed.

▼ Feeding

We've already incorporated food into our solo play in the boot camp section, so why not use it for the next duet? Your top could give you a "grapefruit blow job" (wait for someone to do it to you or read up on the method in "The Gimmick Blow Job" for tops on page 93), while you satisfy his sweet tooth by literally turning your dick into a candy cane. For example, dip your dick into a fruit smoothie, add sugar or a few sprinkles, and voilà: a sticky treat for your top. There are hundreds of possible variations. You can feed your top a new flavor every day.

▼ Plug Job

This can be a favor you do yourself, or a special surprise for your partner. In either case, if the blow job bottom wears a butt plug in his ass while his partner sucks him off, it's a hot invitation to a bonus round and extended play. If the roles are clearly defined in your relationship, you can use this to blow the signal for a reassessment of your respective roles and maybe even a new era. If your lover takes a liking to making your plug vibrate while he sucks you off, it's only a small step to following it up with a rimming session. But it's quite enough for you to start the vibrations yourself.

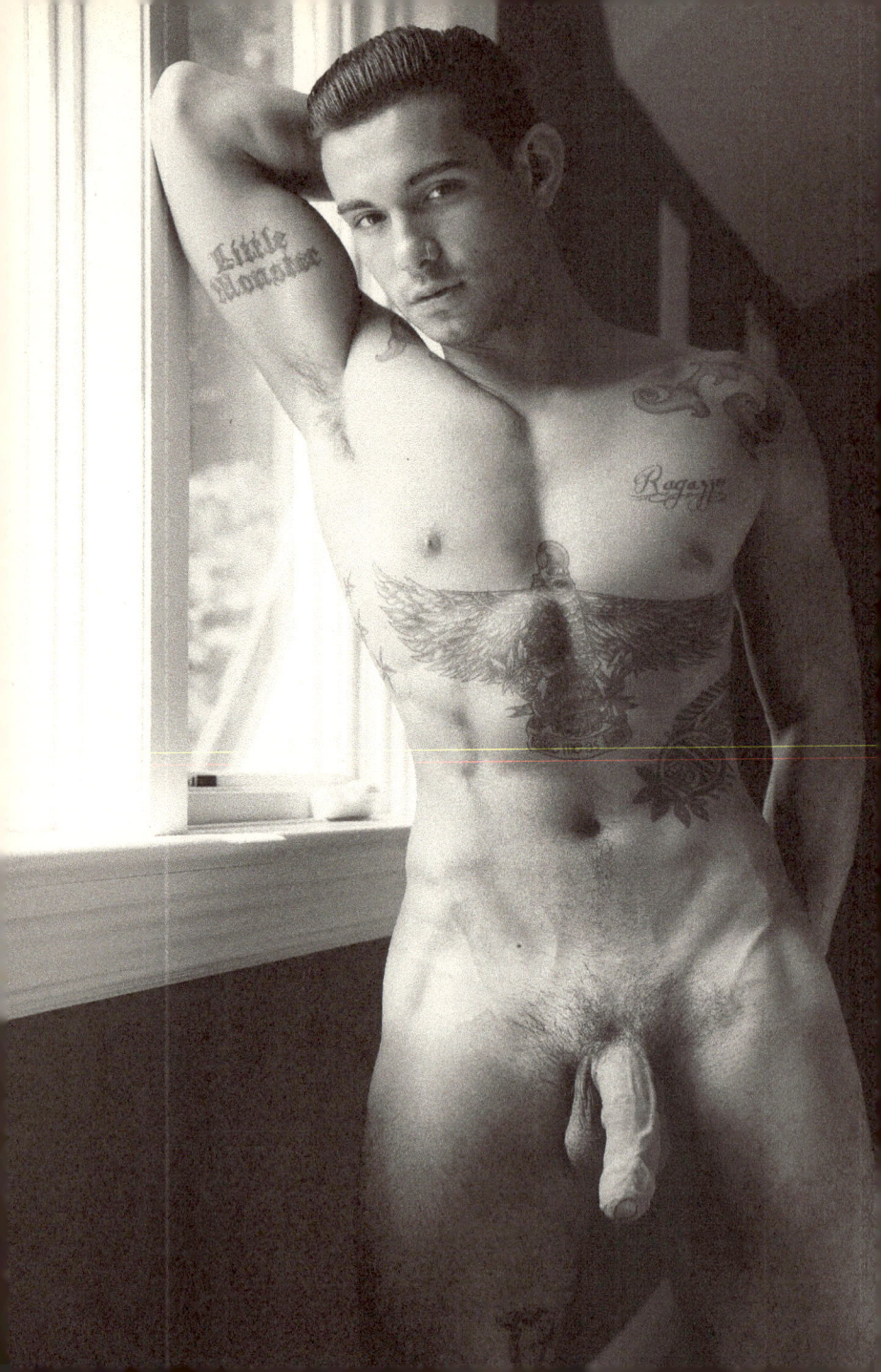

Interview with CockyBoys Blow Job Bottom Ricky Roman: "Good Blow Job Artists Never Quit"

For the blow job man of the world, Ricky Roman and his impressive foreskin are the complete package with extra benefits. Ever since the twenty-four-year-old plunged his boner into a Fleshjack in such a delightful manner at the CockyBoys studio in New York, he has been inundated by fans. Despite this, Ricky has never lost touch with reality. He is amazingly grounded. For one thing, this is due to the fact that, before embarking on his porn career, he took the time to find out what really turns him on—for example: blow job artists with a certain sense of etiquette.

When was your first blow job and what was it like?
I was fifteen, and it happened in a pickup truck. At the time, it felt kind of strange. But it was really hot and it felt incredibly good.

Have you always known you preferred receiving oral sex to giving it?
To be honest, it took a while for me to really enjoy receiving. In my experience, you need to try both roles out for yourself—topping and bottoming. It took a lot of dates before I finally realized I prefer being sucked off.

Your opinion on the following theory: "Oral sex is not just foreplay, it's a whole category of sex in itself"?
I do think that blow jobs are a category in themselves. They aren't quite as clearly defined as anal sex, but you do have to stick to a certain type of etiquette. To start with: no teeth, please!

Do you have any tips for a more intense experience during oral sex?
Communication is key. This is true for every kind of sex and it can lead to a more intense experience during oral sex. I really like praising my partners, telling them what makes them special if they're doing a good job. I also want them to tell me what turns them on about sucking my dick, or just how hot it is for them.

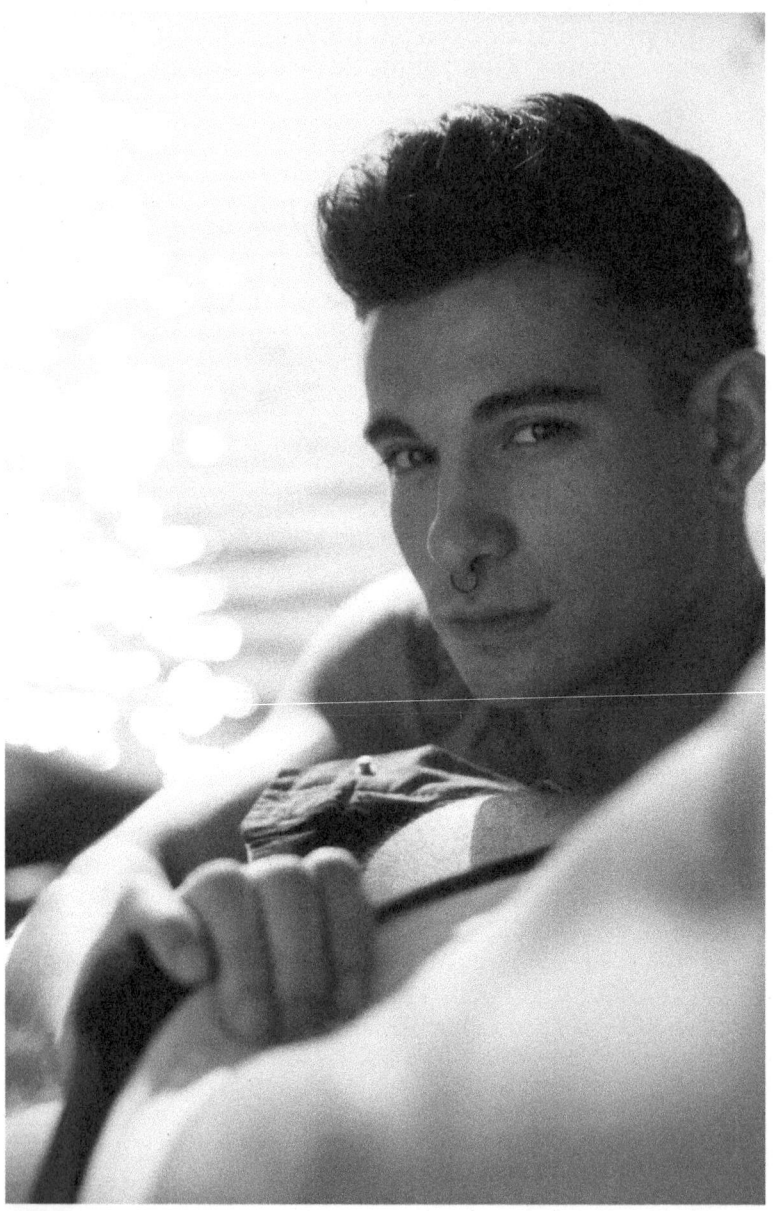

What makes a man a good blow job artist?
Really good blow job artists are careful and conscientious with their technique. They don't scrape their teeth along my cock shaft. They slobber all over my boner and use a lot of spit to get it really wet. They use their hands from time to time to add stimulation. But most importantly, they have stamina; they don't quit until I've ejaculated deep inside their throats or on their faces.

What do you like best about oral sex?
You can suck my dick anywhere, at any time of the day, as long as it's convenient. I don't care if I'm sitting down or standing up.

And the other way round? What constitutes a real turn-off?
Any kind of bad "performance" can be a turn-off—not sucking hard enough, sucking too hand, relying on your hands too much. It also depends on the situation.

What's the biggest challenge for a blow job bottom?
Again, that's a question of how I feel at the time. Sometimes a blow job isn't enough to get me to orgasm. But that also has something to do with how much I need it.

How can one desensitize an oversensitive dick for hard oral sex?
There isn't really a technique for this. You need a lot of experience to control that kind of thing. And that takes time. So you need to take your time.

Can you tell if a man is good at giving oral sex just by looking at him?
No. You can't judge a book by its cover. A sensual mouth doesn't make a guy a top notch blow job artist.

Is there such a thing as a mouth that's "too small"?
I've never come across one myself.

Apart from the blow job itself, what makes oral sex exciting?
As I'm uncircumcised, I like having my foreskin sucked or even nibbled. It's also important for a good blow job to involve my balls, i.e. by massaging them.

Your most memorable blow job up till now...
... Wasn't the blow job itself, it was the man who gave it to me. This guy was completely obsessed with giving oral sex. His technique was incredible, he could really talk dirty and he got me to shoot one load after the next.

Have you ever had an accident during a blow job?
One of my ex-boyfriends overdid it once. Instead of gurgling and gagging, he suddenly started throwing up. Fortunately, he managed to spit my dick out first, so it didn't get on me.

What are your views on the fetishization of "facials" (cumming in someone's face) and swallowing semen?
Where I like to cum depends on my mood. And on my partner. After all, he has to enjoy it too. If he tells me to cum on his face, that's what I'll do.

True or false: "There aren't enough cocksuckers in the world of gay men"?
Trust me, there are plenty of cocksuckers out there. You just need to find out where they're all hiding.

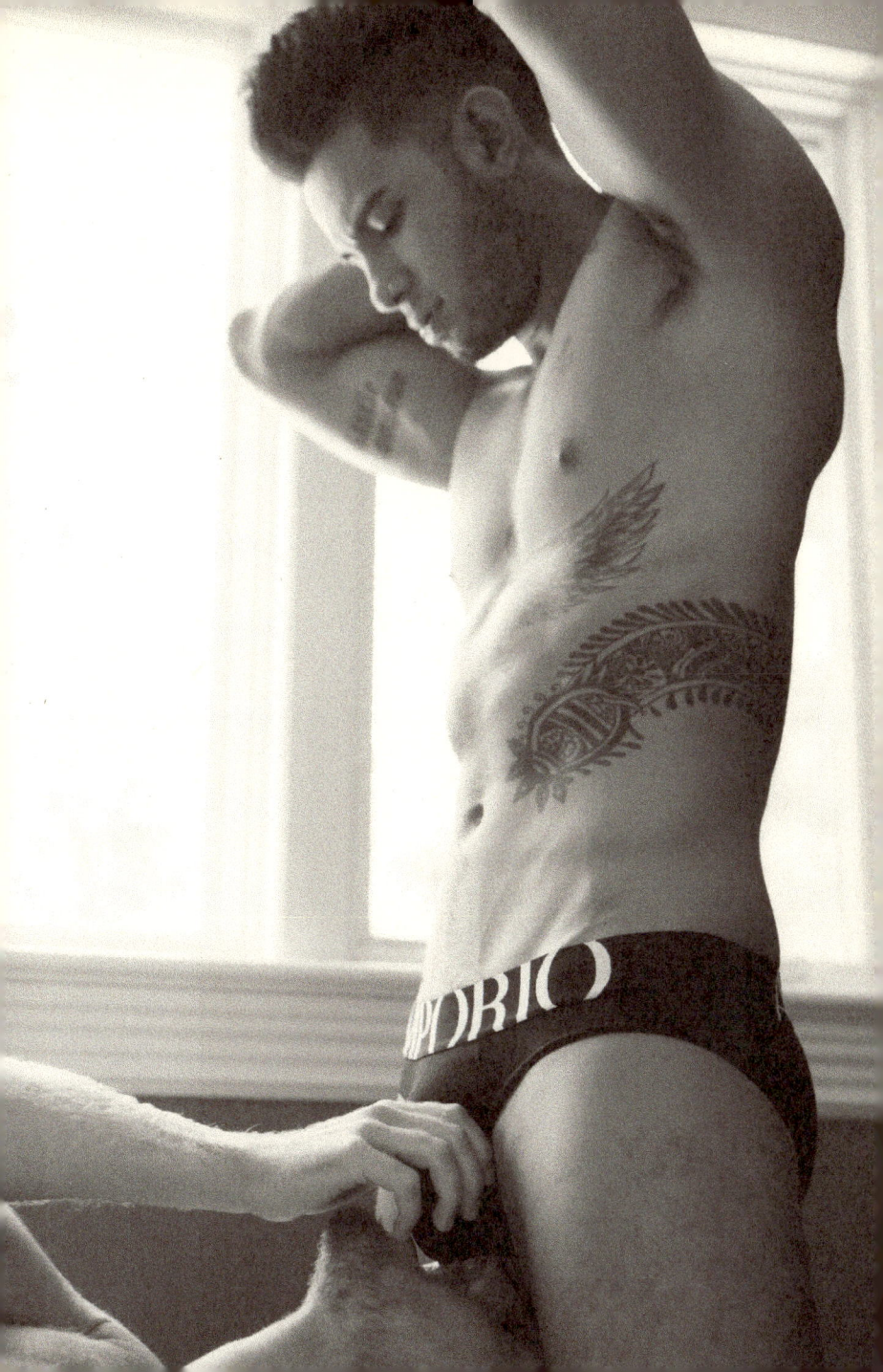

Bonus Material: Blow Job Gimmicks for Bottoms

▼ The Portable Hole

If you're traveling or out in the wild and can't live without a glory hole for your partner to stick his dick through, you can order a "Glory Hole to go" from the website of the same name. You can also use the website as an instruction manual for building your own. With a little technical ingenuity, you can easily build this simple construction out of a frame with a length of fabric with a hole in the middle attached to it.

▼ Cock Rings

We've already gone into using your fingers to produce the "cock ring effect" in the "Equipment" chapter, but there's nothing like the original version. These (metal, plastic, or leather) rings are placed around the root of the penis and prevent the blood from flowing back out of the erectile tissue once it's erect. This makes your boner especially thick, firm, and sensitive. It's an asset for both yourself and your lover. Cock rings should not be worn for more than an hour at a time.

▼ Camcorder

Nearly everyone has one of these gimmicks: the camcorder on your smartphone. You can use this to make your own simple and spontaneous private porn movies. Once you've finished filming, you can decide for yourself whether it's for your own use only or whether you want to upload it to the "amateur" category of one of the relevant video portals. In any case, your partner will make an extra special effort as soon as he feels the stern eye

> **With a little technical ingenuity, you can build your own "Glory Hole to Go."**

of the camera on him. One important point, however: if your lover doesn't want to be filmed during sex, please respect this. And if you do upload the video to the Internet, check with him first.

▼ Tattoos & Piercings

It takes some courage and a lot of willpower, but if you do decide to get a tattoo on your dick, you can be certain of the eternal respect of the entire gay world. Although a tattoo won't have any effect on how a blow job feels once it's healed, it will transform your entire blow job experience. If only because you'll be able to attract an entirely new following. The same applies to piercings, such as the Prince Albert or the Ampallang (right through the glans). If you have the latter, make sure there are no sharp edges that might scratch your partner's throat.

> *Tattoos will transform your entire blow job experience.*

▼ Belts, Ties, Collars

Suit and tie wearers swear by it, as of course do pet players who take their tops out for walks on the end of a leash. "Putting on the reins" involves placing the "rein" around the back of your lover's neck and using it to pull his head, gently at first, then more firmly if necessary, down onto your boner. Warning: please do not put a noose around anybody's neck! It is far too dangerous.

▼ Water, Water Everywhere

Blow jobs and watersports can be easily combined. If you're not into piss but you do enjoy a mess, you can make a big splash with water or other drinks. Spit into your partner's mouth from above, hawk a loogie on him, or stick him in the shower... Anything goes, the less inhibited you are the better. As long as you stick to waterproof surroundings.

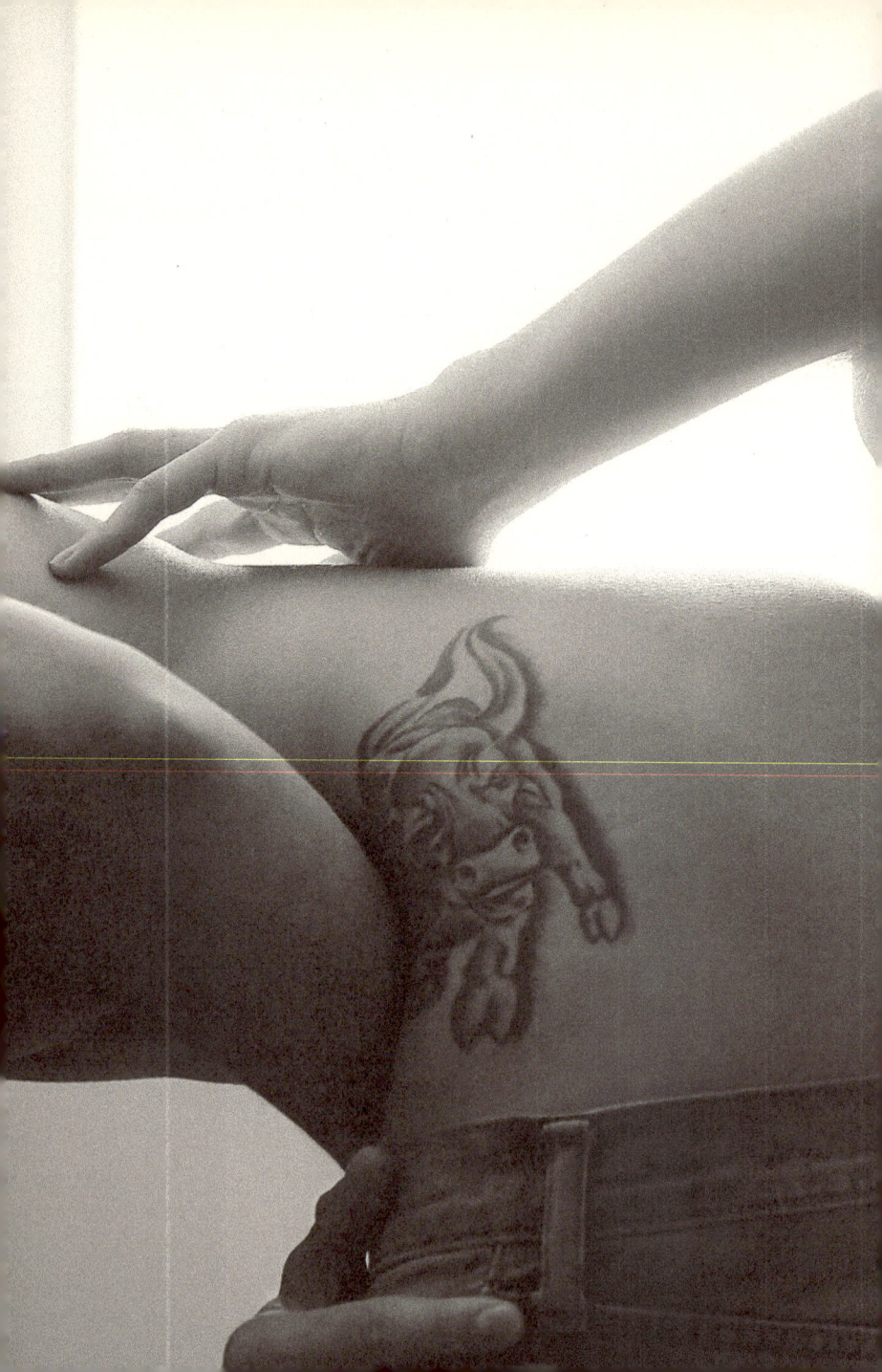

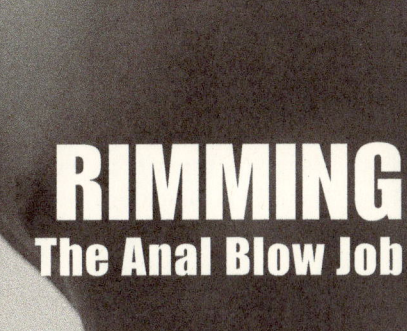

Rimming

From Blow Job to Rim Job

During the first meeting about this book, I got a few funny looks when I said I was going to include a chapter on rimming. But it makes complete sense, right? Not only is the rim job the logical continuation of the blow job, it also has an important place in the range of oral possibilities—and should definitely be included in a book with the subheading "Everything You Need to Know About Oral Sex." So much for the explanation, now let's move on to the substance.

Eating ass is admittedly quite a different activity to sucking dick. It's not about capacity, gag reflexes or opening your mouth, but instead involves skillful handiwork and even more skillful deployment of your tongue, your lower lip and occasionally your nose. It's quite helpful to keep this chapter separate from the fixed categories "top" and "bottom." Because even if the same categories we used for the blow job also apply here (the top does the rimming, the bottom gets rimmed), both participants' functions are reversed at this point. Especially because rimming is, as a rule, undertaken in preparation to anal sex, and the blow job bottom's role switches to that of an anal top. Apart from that, we can generally divide the course of a rimming session into the following steps.

Step 1 – Prep phase: All asses are different, so you will need to take stock of the situation prior to every rim job. Are you gazing into a deep ass crack with voluptuous cheeks or is it one of those boney asses where you can see his anus the moment he opens his legs? These anatomical conditions will determine how easy it will be to place your mouth where you want it: on his anus.

Step 2 – Licking it open: Place your hands on either side of his butt cheeks, stick your thumbs inside the crack and open it up around his hole. Now stick out your tongue and give his butt crack a swipe from top to bottom. Then turn your attention to his anus. Employ the same circling motions you used while giving a blow job to trace around the sphincter with the tip of your tongue. Keep doing that until your partner has gotten used to it. Then: push the tip of your tongue deeper into the hole! After that, start from the beginning again—until it's all nice and wet and his hole has opened up.

Step 3 – Feeling your way: Push your index finger into his hole as far as you can. Confirm whether your partner likes it. Then slowly move your finger back and forth. Hint: Make sure your fingernails are short and smooth to prevent injuries!

Step 4 – Dive in: Following the finger exercise, you should be able to pull the sphincter open further than before. This gives your tongue the chance to rotate inside the sensitive membranes of the rectum. You're now ready to dive right into the rim job.

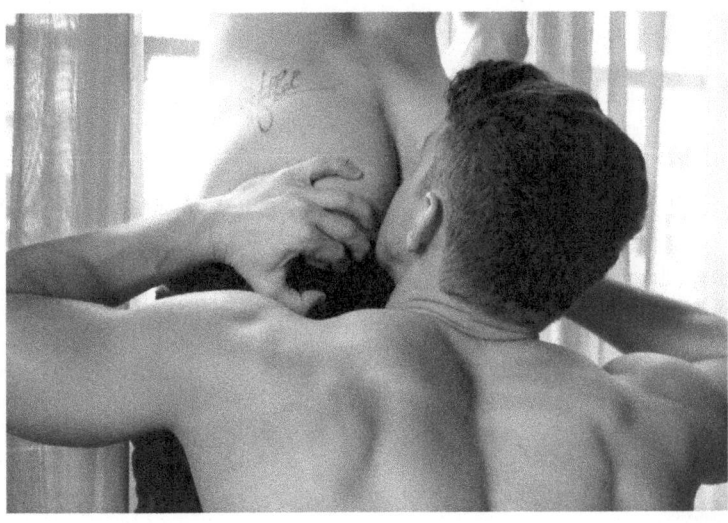

Ass-Eating Deluxe—Five Rimming Tips

▼ Anilingus & Co.

"Ana" as in "anal" and "lingus" as in "lick"—this is the Latin term for tossing a guy's salad. In some ways, analingus is closely related to its sister discipline, cunnilingus. The latter won't be of much interest to most of my readers, but that doesn't mean we can't take a few tips from the muff divers. Three cunnilingus tips for your anus.

Training: A good rim job is even more dependent on having a quick and agile tongue than a blow job. So you will need to train your tongue. You can either practice sticking it out in front of a mirror, taking the stone out of a peach and licking out the hole, or invest in a "Lick This" app that sends instructions to your smartphone on how to lick your touchscreen. It's literally a matter of taste.

Shifting the action: As all cunning linguists and their partners know, if your tongue gets tired, your neck muscles can be a first-class replacement. "Huh?" I hear you say, and then: "Oh, right." If you can't send your tongue darting out in every direction, just stick it in the hole and waggle your head around. This has a similar effect to moving your tongue around, especially if your partner is already fired up.

Patience: Women are no more fussy about sex then men are, that's just a silly rumor; but they are a lot more sensitive when you talk to them. Especially when the conversation turns to how they like having their vaginas licked. Which is why every guide to cunnilingus will stress the importance of patience, tenderness, and care. You should apply these virtues to eating ass, if only to be aware of the fact that the anus and the realms that lie behind it are a lot more sensitive than your average dick.

▼ Cleanliness

Shit! If we're talking about the joys of anal sex, there's no way of getting around this crappy issue. Although that's easily solved. As long as the bottom is more or less aware of his body and has taken a shower recently, this goes a long way to reducing the danger of the top getting shit up his nose. In certain situations, however, it is only fair to take a pass on having your ass licked. These include:

- If you realize you're about to drop a load.
- If you haven't washed your butt for more than a day.
- If you have diarrhea.
- If you suffer from bowel leakage due to medical issues (such as hemorrhoids). Wipe your butt with toilet paper to check or... check your underpants for skid marks.

If you're into scat (shit play), please don't do this if you haven't agreed on it with your partner beforehand. This preference isn't widely shared, which is why your partner is far more likely to react in horror to a stinky brown surprise than delight. Please reserve surprises for those men of whom you are absolutely sure that they will appreciate them. To prepare for a scheduled rimming session, the bottom should proceed as follows:

> *You can easily avoid the top getting shit up his nose.*

- Get yourself an anal douche and use it two hours beforehand.
- If you do take a dump in between, use a wet-wipe to clean yourself and wait for at least two hours.
- If you don't feel clean, go to the toilet or take a shower.
- Don't go on a date with a very full stomach. Especially as it will also make you sluggish.

▼ Safer Rimming

Eating ass is a relative safe activity for the guy getting eaten, but the other guy is at risk for a number of infections. Again, awareness of your own health and sticking to some minimum standards of hygiene can also help prevent accidents. Rimming puts you at a high risk of contracting hepatitis A and B, as these viruses can be easily transmitted via contact with tiny amounts of shit. Bu,: vaccines against hepatitis A and B are available. So take them and cut out the risk of contracting these infections in the first place. Apart from that, always take a close look beforehand! If you spot any pimples, swellings, or sores around your partner's anus, tell him! He may have gonorrhea, herpes, syphilis, or anal warts and not even know it. I know, interrupting a rim job because you suspect an infection is awkward and not terribly sexy. But let's be honest, you owe it to yourself, to your partner, and to your partner's future partners to speak up. If you don't, this can affect not only you, but many other men as well. The diseases I mentioned are transmitted via direct contact with their external symptoms (pimples, swellings, and sores) during a rim job.

Interrupting a rim job is awkward and not sexy. But you owe it to yourself.

Now let's talk about HIV. As long as there's no bleeding, you are unlikely to contract HIV via rimming. But if you don't trust your partner's self-assessment or your own eyes, you can always use dental dams (called that because they are commonly used by dentists). These very thin, elastic sheets of latex are placed over your mouth or your partner's anus to prevent direct contact. They take some getting used to, but that's what we all used to say about condoms as well. So if you feel safer with a dam, why not?

▼ Techniques

Only individual experience will tell you what tongue moves work best for both of you, but for guaranteed satisfaction, you should at least try all out the most common techniques. Here they are!

Anal probe: First of all, check how far you can go. That's how you start. This means, point your tongue and dip it into his hole as far as you can. Then you can either move it back and forth for a tongue-fuck, or stay down below and try out some of the other techniques.

Circles: Circling the tip of your tongue around his anus as part of foreplay is one thing, doing the same thing inside his rectum quite another. This requires concentration and sensitivity. Check in with your lover from time to time to make sure he's enjoying it.

Ping-pong: Once the sphincter muscles have relaxed enough for you to pull them apart with your thumbs, you can make your tongue dart back and forth from one side of his anus to the other, like a ping-pong ball. Whether you go up and down or side to side is up to you.

Slalom: Swiping your tongue along his ass crack from top to bottom is a great way to relax and prepare both of you for the following rimming action, and it can be expanded to create a tongue slalom.

Sucking: While you're licking his anus, purse your lips and suck it as if you were kissing it—you have to try this!

▼ Short & Sweet

Rim job tops should also be well-groomed. Beards are the major issue. Not everyone enjoys the prickling sensation of beard stubble on the sensitive skin of his anus. Hair regrowth can give you a chin like a cheese grater, which may also irritate the skin. Keep that beard trimmed. And once again: your nails should be short, clean, and free of rips and tears before your fingers go anywhere near your partner's asshole.

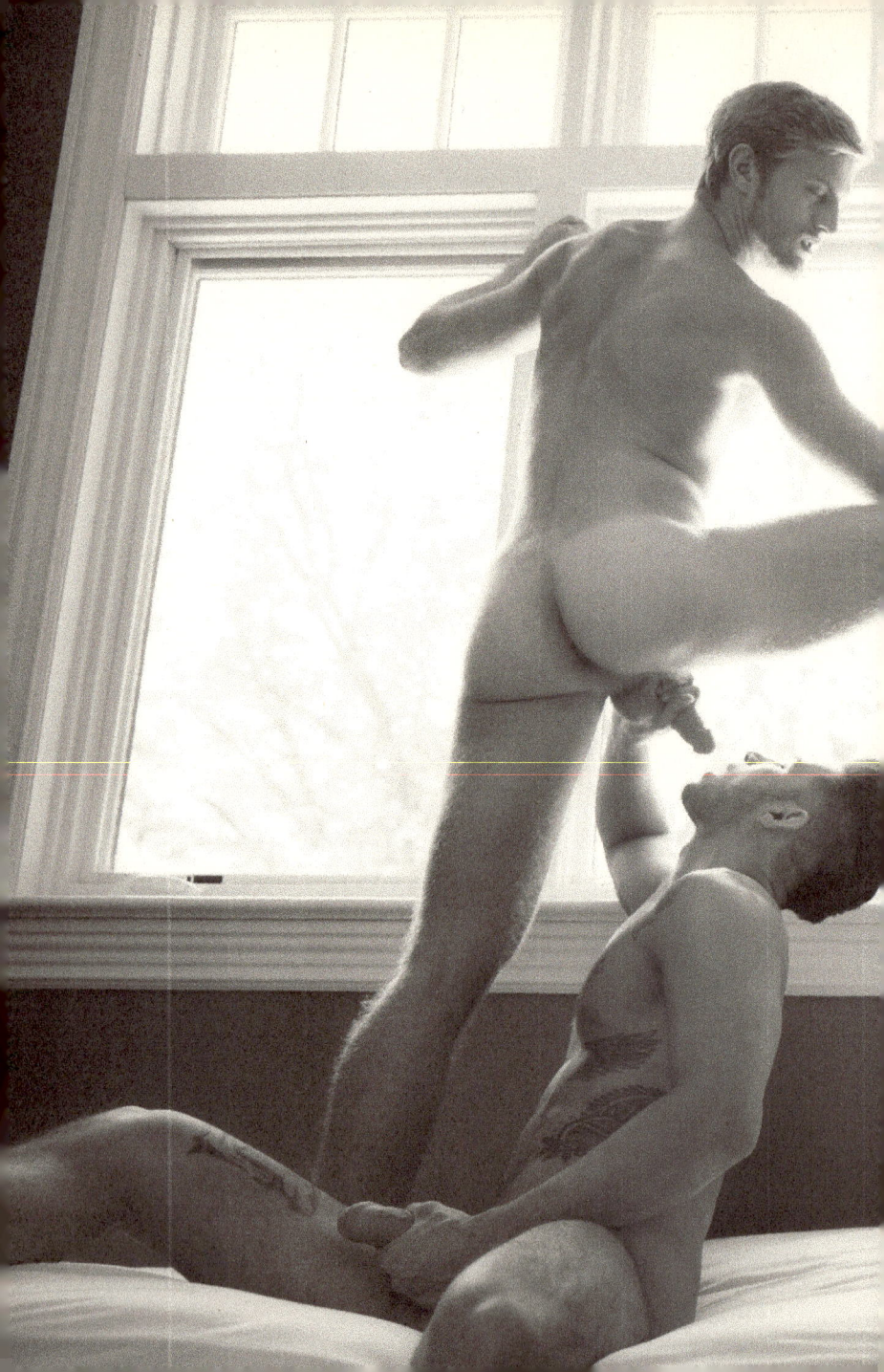

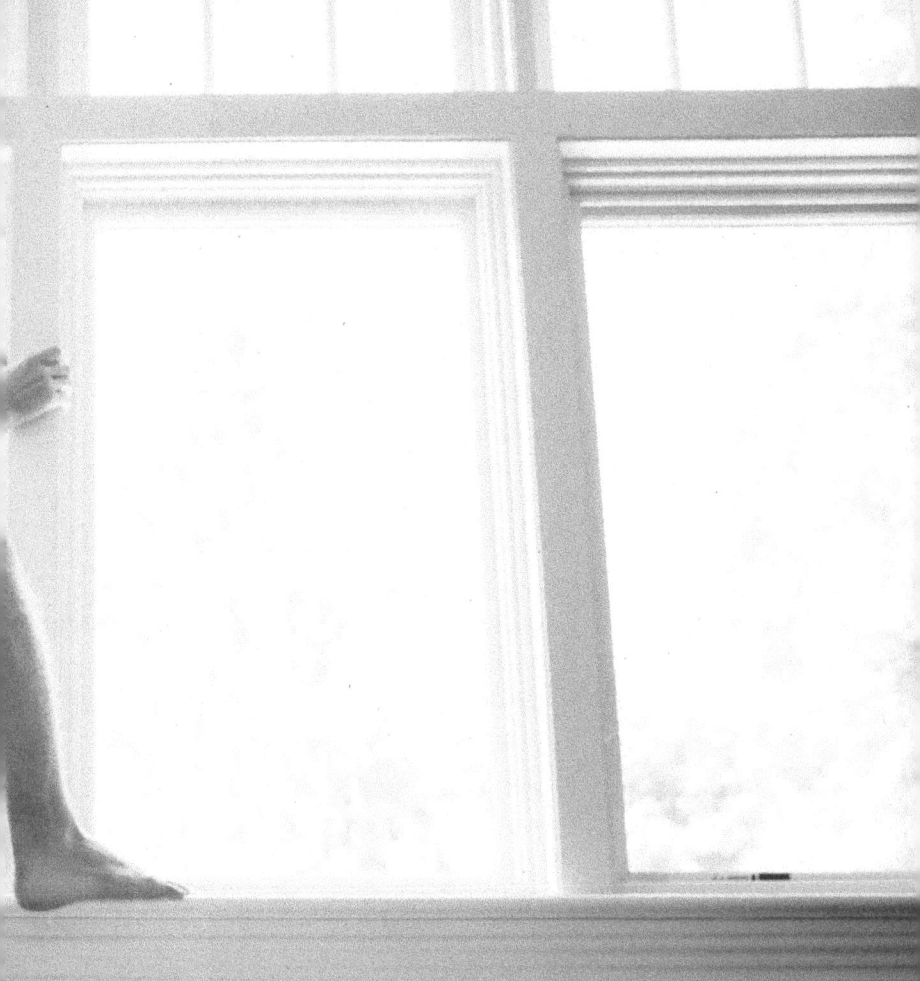

SWALLOWING
Competitive Cum-Guzzling

_____Swallowing

Conspicuous Consumption—A New Phenomenon?

I was recently discussing the new semen-hype with a friend of mine when I asked him "When did the whole swallowing thing start?" He answered, "You know, it was never really over."

Let me explain: I am now in my mid-thirties, which makes me part of a generation that grew up with the awareness that swallowing semen was really dangerous and could give you HIV. So you just didn't do it. In my case, this also applied to relationships. We jerked off onto each other's faces and smeared the stuff around, we even licked our own juice off each other's bodies, but I have never knelt in front of my partner while he panted his way towards orgasm with my mouth open and my tongue sticking out. This may have something to do with the fact that all my relationships were with people who pretty soon agreed that monogamy was just an illusion. And if I did get a drop or two in my mouth, I always spat it out quickly and rinsed my mouth out. End of story! This approach put a stop to any semen-swallowing on a grand scale from the very outset. Maybe it also prevented me from developing a taste for the stuff.

The abovementioned friend is fifteen years older than me. He came out just before the AIDS crisis knocked the gay community into a state of shock and terror, and still remembers a time before that. He caught the virus in the late nineties. Therapy was already available then. Which means he never really suffered from any terrible medical complications as a result of HIV. On the other hand, his sex life came to an abrupt standstill for a few months following his diagnosis. He was unable to imagine having sex with other men without being afraid. Even condoms couldn't take away the fear of infecting other people with the virus. But time heals all wounds. His fears abated after a while, he started going out again and at some point, he discovered the world of positive parties. While I was still cutting a swathe through the dating and darkroom scene with the firm belief that hardly anyone was into swallowing, he had cheerfully taken it up again.

Which takes us to the present day. Now that medical professionals are certain that a person infected with HIV on antiretroviral therapy and with completely suppressed viremia is no longer infectious and especially since the development of PrEP (Pre-Exposure Prophylaxis = HIV-medication for HIV-negatives for the purposes of immunization), fucking without a condom has become more generally acceptable and swallowing is no longer restricted to positive parties, but has returned to the mainstream. Apart from the fact that, thinking back, I do in fact recall a couple of situations where a guy gave me a blow job in a darkroom and, when I dutifully announced "I'm about to cum!" did not react by spitting out my dick but instead, dug his fingers into my ass to plug me into him more tightly until I ejaculated. It even happened to me twice with the same guy. That was his thing, I guess. I didn't recognize him the second time until he used the same method. The first time, I tried arguing with him, but this time, I just said "Are you sure you want this?" He nodded and disappeared.

Why am I telling you all this? To explain my reservations on the subject of swallowing. Ultimately, ingesting semen puts you at a lower risk of catching HIV or another infection than fucking without a condom, but the risk is still there. Especially as you can never know for sure whether your partner has suppressed viremia or is on PrEP. So before I go into any specific cum-guzzling rituals, I would like to emphasize that this is the least safe form of oral sex. If you don't want to run the risk of infection, you might want to consider the alternatives I have added to every practice. This applies not only to HIV-negative readers. After all, you can catch syphilis, chlamydia or gonorrhea just as easily via swallowing.

Seven Cum Play Techniques, Seven Alternatives

▼ Swallowing

Many people are grossed out at first, but get used to it after a while: standard cum swallowing, commonly referred to as plain "swallowing" in most dating forums. Whether you prefer deep-throating the stuff straight into your gullet or target practice, where your open mouth is the target—the variations are endless. If you do it because you're really turned on by the taste and consistency, you'll want to keep doing it (in which case you should try and find non-infectious partners), but if you just force yourself to do it because you think it will make you look cool or be accepted, please remember that good sex is a result of self-determination, not peer pressure.
Alternative: Self-Feeding Yoga

▼ Snowballing

"Snowballing" refers to a technique where the blow job top catches his partner's jizz in his mouth and then spits it into his partner's mouth. Who then spits it back into the top's mouth. And then gets it back again. And so on. Devotion plays a large role in this highly symbolic game.
Alternative: Who says it has to be semen? It's just those people who ascribe mythical qualities to their sperm and see it as an expression of virility, audacity and (this one's especially dumb) "naturalness." The mental and emotional significance of this is understandable, but largely overrated. Spitting coke, water, beer or (if you really have to use bodily fluids) spit and piss is just as much fun.

▼ Felching

If you're going to suck your own semen out of your partner's asshole (which is what felching means), you will generally have to cum inside him without a condom first. Which makes it more of a fucking category than a blow job category. But it is definitely a variation

of rimming, which is why I mention it here. Not to mention the fact that some experts will jerk off into a glass and use a syringe to squirt their cum into their partner's asshole before sucking it out again.
Alternative: The sex industry never misses a trick. You can choose from a range of white, viscous lubes on the market, all of which have a similar consistency to semen. "Load" by Mister B is just one example.

▼ Gokkun

It sounds like something teenagers would do on a dare, but it is actually an entire porn genre in Japan. You get as many guys as possible to jerk off into a glass and then someone has to drink the entire contents. It's like an advanced version of the soggy biscuit game. As getting enough men together to fill an entire glass with semen presents quite a logistical challenge for one person, one strategy can be to freeze a whole bunch of semen until you've collected enough. That doesn't make it any more fresh, but it does take us straight to the alternative version.
Alternative: Mythical qualities aside—if you're allowed to cheat anyway by freezing the stuff, then you can just take it one step further and freeze your own juice. It doesn't taste any different.

▼ Self-Feeding Yoga

If you've always dreamed of having semen squirted into your mouth, why not start with your own? With just a little willpower and agility, most men will be able to raise their legs up into the "candle" position, then throw them back behind their heads in a sort of half-backward somersault and hit themselves in the face. The goal is clearly to ejaculate into your own mouth. It's a bit wobbly and uncomfortable, but it does have the benefit of allowing you to feed yourself with your own semen. As this requires you to ejaculate first, your affinity for swallowing will have to pass the post-orgasmic agility test.
Alternative: Not strictly necessary in this case, but you can of course just jerk off onto your stomach, wipe it off, and then lick your fingers clean.

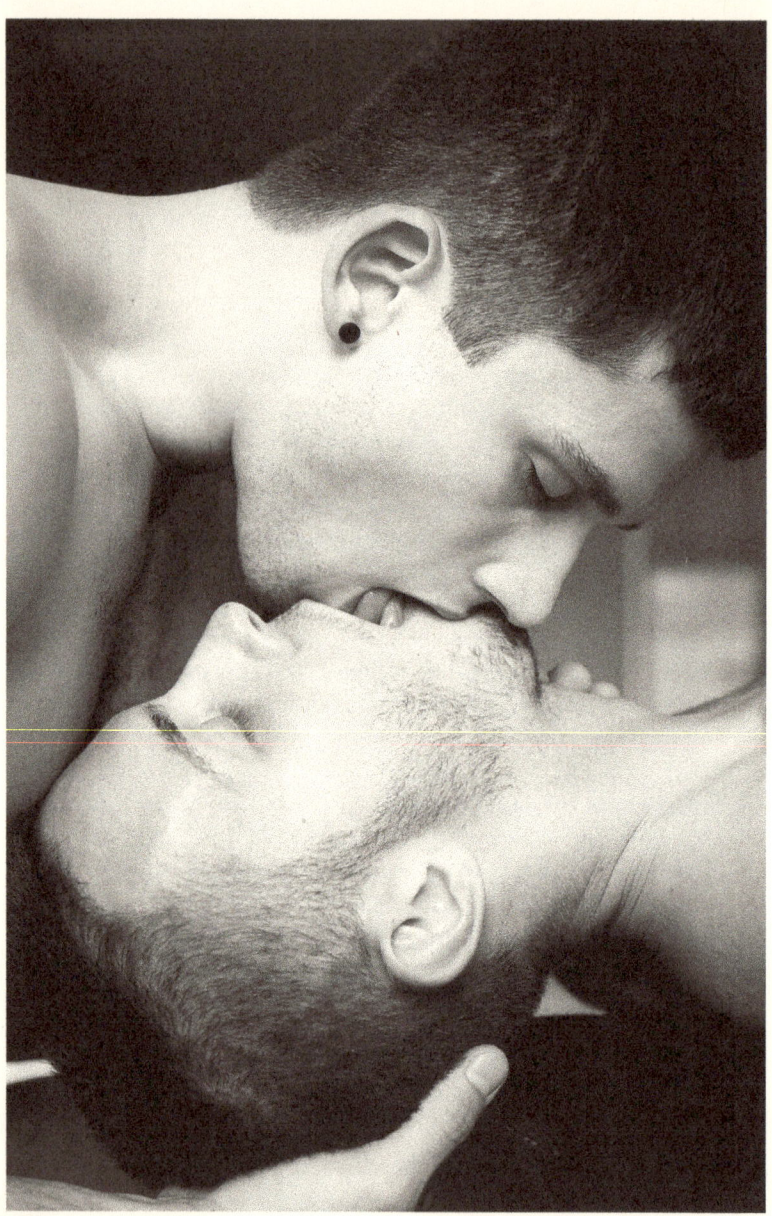

▼ Chain Reaction

A pleasure shared is a pleasure doubled... And tripled... And quadrupled... And so on. "Cum Swapping" is a group sex variation on snowballing. As in the good old telephone game of your childhood, you and your partners pass each other's semen from mouth to mouth: an activity that can grow to assume positively ritualistic proportions. Especially if you do it in a BDSM context, following your Master's orders. This is another type of psychological kick, one that plays with the gene-carrying function of semen.

Alternative: If rituals hold such as strong fascination for you, attending communion might be an option. Just joking. Sorry, I couldn't resist. Otherwise, the same alternatives to snowballing work here as well: Try swapping beer, coke, or piss instead.

▼ Semen Doping

Ginseng, goji berries and garlic are all said to increase sperm production, giving you especially copious ejaculations. Is that true? Who cares? As long as you believe in it. Many people do not, which is why the natural remedy industry has developed a range of pills with names like Volume Pills or Spermomax that promise to deliver larger "loads." Gay porn star Spencer Quest has endorsed one of these products, saying that "Jaculex not only works, it works wonders." Well maybe it does. But don't tell me this has anything to do with being "natural."

Alternative: Just abstain from ejaculating for a week. Boring, I know. But in this case, the size of your load will indeed correlate with the intensity of your orgasm.

Shut Your Mouth—Closing Remarks

Blowing, rimming, swallowing! Topping, bottoming, theorizing! That pretty much covers the entire spectrum of oral pleasure and now it's time for all of us to fan out and test our new-found knowledge in bedrooms, cruising areas and sex cubs all over the world. Now some of you might say you would have liked to learn more. About oral double penetration, for example. Or about piss play. Or about countries where oral sex is illegal. Let me respond to these in the same order: double penetration may involve a higher level of difficulty and coordination, but ultimately it is governed by the same rules as a simple blow job. It does not require its own chapter. With regard to piss play, we have mentioned it in passing, but watersports are really a category of their own rather than a variety of oral sex. And the countries where oral sex is a crime? Ever since Singapore lifted the ban on oral sex in 2007, these no longer exist in the comprehensive sense of the term. In the narrower sense of course, they do. For guys. In countries with a ban on all gay sexual activity, this rule obviously applies to oral sex as well. There are still over seventy of these countries. Most of them are in Africa or the Middle East with the most draconian punishments (the death penalty) found in Nigeria, Brunei, and Iran. Discussing the rights of gay men on a global scale in a book about blow jobs is probably taking things a little too far, which is why I don't feel that this is the right place for a proper discussion of these topics. However, the subject does of cause help us see our own privileged position in an entirely different light. At least in those parts of the world where this book will probably be read, we are extremely lucky to be able to engage with sexual practices such as blow jobs in such a hedonistic and, in the best sense of the word, shameless form. And to be left with unanswered questions once we've finished. And to be brave enough to ask these questions. And to be able to find our own answers. In thousands of bedrooms, cruising areas and sex clubs around the world. We've come full circle. Good luck and, above all, have fun!

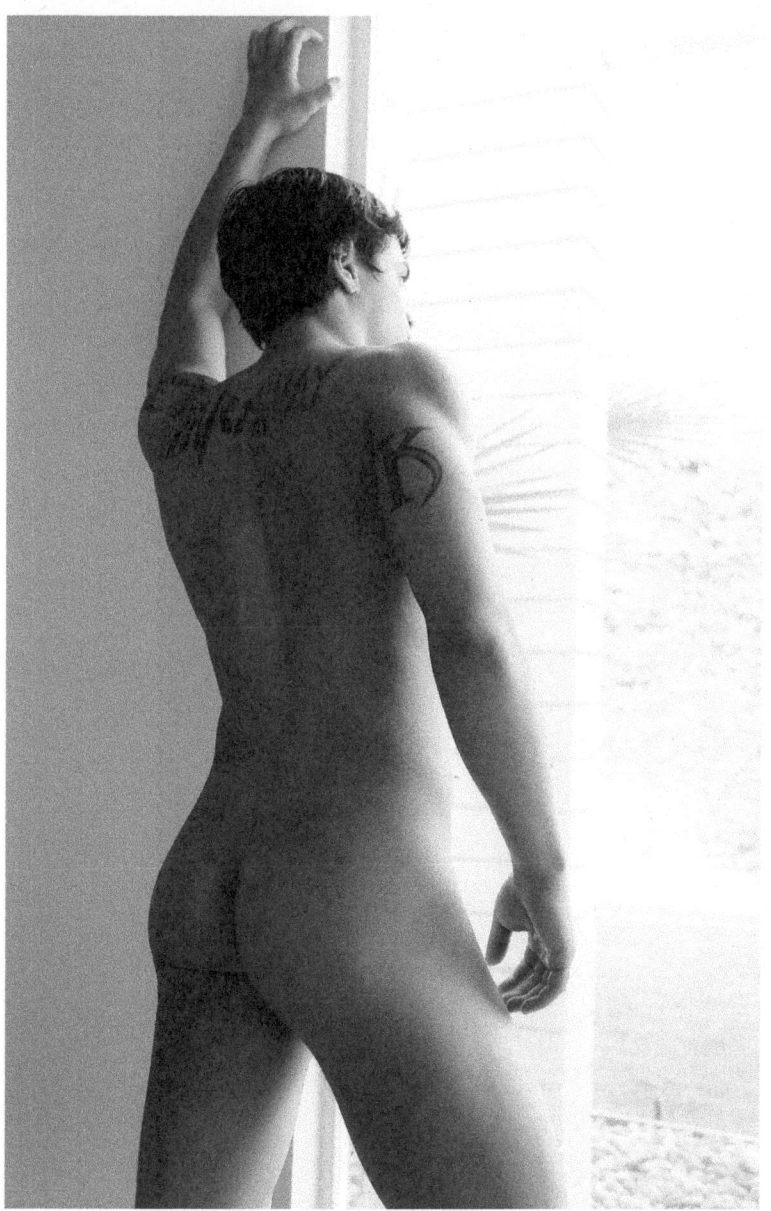

Model: Jake Bass

COCKYBOYS.COM